The Guide to Clinical Preventive Services

2014

Recommendations of the U.S. Preventive Services Task Force

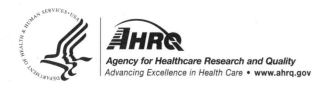

AHRQ

Agency for Healthcare Research and Quality
Advancing Excellence in Health Care • www.ahrq.gov

Foreword

Since 1998, the Agency for Healthcare Research and Quality (AHRQ) has convened the U.S. Preventive Services Task Force (USPSTF)—an independent, volunteer panel of national experts in prevention and evidence-based medicine. The Task Force makes recommendations to help primary care clinicians and patients decide together whether a preventive service is right for a patient's needs.

AHRQ staff provide scientific and administrative support for the Task Force, and assist in disseminating its findings and recommendations to key audiences. In that role, we are pleased to make *The Guide to Clinical Preventive Services 2014* available to those who seek to ensure that their patients receive the highest quality clinical preventive services.

I am gratified that AHRQ has been able to support the USPSTF in its efforts to engage the public and to ensure that its processes are transparent. Most notably, all Task Force draft materials are now available for public comment online at www. USPreventiveServicesTaskForce.org.

Previous iterations of the USPSTF *Guide to Clinical Preventive Services* are used around the Nation to provide appropriate and effective preventive care. The *Guide* is designed to be user-friendly for practicing clinicians. In addition, the *Guide* lists resources that clinicians can use to educate their patients on appropriate preventive services, such as *Stay Healthy* brochures and MyHealthfinder (see Appendixes). Also included are brief descriptions of and links to tools that health care professionals can use to improve their practice, including the electronic Preventive Services Selector (ePSS) and the National Guideline Clearinghouse (see Appendixes).

As more information becomes available to clinicians and patients alike, AHRQ's goal is to help improve patients' health and well-being, and contribute to better health outcomes for the Nation overall.

Richard Kronick, Ph.D.
Director
Agency for Healthcare Research and Quality

Preface

The U.S. Preventive Services Task Force (USPSTF) is mandated by Congress to conduct rigorous reviews of scientific evidence to create evidence-based recommendations for preventive services that may be provided in the primary care setting.

Since its inception, the USPSTF has made and maintained recommendations on dozens of clinical preventive services that are intended to prevent or reduce the risk for heart disease, cancer, infectious diseases, and other conditions and events that impact the health of children, adolescents, adults, and pregnant women. The *Guide to Clinical Preventive Services 2014* includes both new and updated recommendations released from 2004-2014 in a brief, easily usable format meant for use at the point of patient care. The most up-to-date version of the recommendations, as well as the complete USPSTF recommendation statements, are available along with their supporting scientific evidence at www.USPreventiveServicesTaskForce.org.

Recommendations for preventive care have evolved over time as it has become widely recognized that some "preventive" services were not actually beneficial. Individual health care providers, professional organizations, integrated health systems, insurers (both private and public), as well as groups crafting health quality measures and national health objectives, have recognized the need to carefully balance potential benefits and harms using the highest quality of evidence, and have adopted the recommendations of the Task Force. The primary audience for the USPSTF's work remains primary care clinicians, and the recommendations are now considered by many to provide definitive standards for preventive services. The work of the USPSTF is recognized by the Patient Protection and Affordable Care Act. Under the law, preventive services with a Task Force grade of A or B must be covered without cost-sharing (e.g., copayment or deductible) under new health insurance plans or policies.

In the last several years, the USPSTF has increased the transparency of its work, and these efforts have gained additional momentum in view of the enhanced importance of the recommendations under the new law. Public comments are welcomed at multiple points in the development of each recommendation to encourage additional input from experts, advocates and other stakeholders to help the Task Force craft relevant and clear recommendation statements. However, the USPSTF remains committed to evaluating evidence free from the influence of politics, special interests, and advocacy.

As the science around clinical practice guideline development has evolved, USPSTF methods continue to evolve as well. The Procedure Manual, which can be found on the USPSTF Web site, details the most updated version of the process for evaluating the quality and strength of the evidence for a service, determining the net health benefit (benefit minus harms) associated with the service, and judging the level of certainty that providing these services will be beneficial in primary care. We continue to explore the appropriate use of mathematical modeling to help fill research gaps regarding the ages at which to start and stop providing a service, and at what time intervals. In addition, we are committed to improving the communication of our recommendations to a broader audience, including patients and policymakers.

The letter grade linked to each recommendation reflects both the magnitude of net benefit and the strength and certainty of the evidence supporting the provision of a specific preventive service. These grades translate to practice guidance for clinicians:

- Discuss services with "A" and "B" recommendation grades with eligible patients and offer them as a priority.

- Discourage the use of services with "D" recommendation grades unless there are unusual additional considerations.

- Give lower priority to services with "C" recommendation grades; they need not be provided unless there are individual considerations in favor of providing the service.

- Help patients understand the uncertainty surrounding services with "I" (insufficient evidence) statements, which reflect the conclusion that the evidence is insufficient to determine net benefit. The Clinical Considerations section of each full recommendation statement offers additional guidance.

The USPSTF recognizes that clinical decisions about patients involve more complex considerations than the evidence alone; clinicians should always understand the evidence but individualize decisionmaking to the specific patient and situation. The Clinical Considerations section of each USPSTF recommendation statement helps clinicians by offering practical information so they can tailor these recommendations to individual patients.

We strongly encourage clinicians to visit the USPSTF Web site and read the complete recommendation statements for services relevant to their patients. Additional information is available to facilitate the delivery of the highest quality preventive care. For each topic, educational materials have been developed for use with patients and the public. Special materials developed for clinicians are also available on some complex topics, such as prostate and lung cancer screening, along with links to informative Web sites. In addition, the USPSTF Electronic Preventive Services

Selector (ePSS), available via PDA, smart phone, or on the Web at epss.ahrq.gov, allows users to search USPSTF recommendations by patient age and other clinical characteristics.

We hope you find the *Guide to Clinical Preventive Services 2014* to be a useful tool as you care for patients. Based on the best medical evidence available, we are confident that by implementing these recommended services, you will help your patients live longer and healthier lives.

Michael L. LeFevre, M.D., M.S.P.H., Chair
Albert L. Siu, M.D., M.S.P.H., Co-Vice Chair
Kirsten Bibbins-Domingo, Ph.D., M.D., M.A.S., Co-Vice Chair
U.S. Preventive Services Task Force

Contents

Clinical Summaries of Recommendations for Children and Adolescents (alphabetical list) 65

*New recommendations released March 2012 to March 2014.

Preventive Services Recommended by the USPSTF

All clinical summaries in this Guide are abridged recommendations. To see the full recommendation statements and recommendations published after March 2014, go to www.USPreventiveServicesTaskForce.org.

The U.S. Preventive Services Task Force (USPSTF) recommends that clinicians discuss these preventive services with eligible patients and offer them as a priority. All these services have received an "A" or a "B" (recommended) grade from the Task Force. Refer to the endnotes for each recommendation for population-specific clinical considerations.

For definitions of all grades used by the USPSTF, see Appendix A (beginning on p. 97). The full listings of all USPSTF recommendations for adults begin on p. 5 and recommendations for children begin on p. 65.

Recommendation	Adults		Special Populations	
	Men	Women	Pregnant Women	Children/Adolescents
Abdominal Aortic Aneurysm, Screening[1]	✓			
Alcohol Misuse Screening and Behavioral Counseling	✓	✓	✓	
Aspirin for the Prevention of Cardiovascular Disease[2]	✓	✓		
Bacteriuria, Screening[3]			✓	
BRCA-Related Cancer in Women, Screening[4]		✓		
Breast Cancer, Preventive Medications[5]		✓		
Breast Cancer, Screening[6]		✓		
Breastfeeding, Counseling[7]		✓	✓	
Cervical Cancer, Screening[8]		✓		
Chlamydial Infection, Screening[9]		✓	✓	
Colorectal Cancer, Screening[10]	✓	✓		
Congenital Hypothyroidism, Screening[11]				✓
Depression in Adults, Screening[12]		✓		
Diabetes Mellitus, Screening[13]	✓	✓		
Falls in Older Adults, Counseling, Preventive Medication, and Other Interventions[14]	✓	✓		

Recommendation	Adults		Special Populations	
	Men	Women	Pregnant Women	Children/Adolescents
Folic Acid Supplementation to Prevent Neural Tube Defects, Preventive Medication[15]		✓		
Gestational Diabetes Mellitus, Screening[16]			✓	
Gonococcal Ophthalmia Neonatorum, Preventive Medication[17]				✓
Gonorrhea, Screening[18]		✓		
Hearing Loss in Newborns, Screening[19]				✓
Hepatitis B Virus Infection in Pregnant Women, Screening[20]			✓	
Hepatitis C Virus Infection in Adults, Screening[21]	✓	✓	✓	✓
High Blood Pressure in Adults, Screening	✓	✓		
HIV Infection, Screening[22]	✓	✓	✓	✓
Intimate Partner Violence and Elderly Abuse, Screening[23]		✓		
Iron Deficiency Anemia, Prevention[24]				
Iron Deficiency Anemia, Screening[25]			✓	
Lipid Disorders in Adults, Screening[26]	✓	✓		
Lung Cancer, Screening[27]	✓	✓		
Major Depressive Disorder in Children and Adolescents, Screening[28]				✓
Obesity in Adults, Screening[29]	✓	✓		
Obesity in Children and Adolescents, Screening[30]				✓
Osteoporosis, Screening[31]		✓		

Section 1: Preventive Services Recommended by the USPSTF *(continued)*

Recommendation	Adults		Special Populations	
	Men	Women	Pregnant Women	Children/Adolescents
Phenylketonuria (PKU), Screening[32]				✓
Sexually Transmitted Infections, Counseling[33]	✓	✓		✓
Sickle Cell Disease in Newborns, Screening[34]				✓
Skin Cancer, Counseling[35]	✓	✓	✓	
Syphilis Infection (Pregnant Women), Screening			✓	
Tobacco Use in Adults, Counseling and Interventions[36]	✓	✓	✓	
Tobacco Use in Children and Adolescents, Primary Care Interventions[37]				✓
Visual Impairment in Children Ages 1 to 5, Screening[38]				✓

[1]One-time screening by ultrasonography in men aged 65 to 75 who have ever smoked.

[2]When the potential harm of an increase in gastrointestinal hemorrhage is outweighed by a potential benefit of a reduction in myocardial infarctions (men aged 45-79 years) or in ischemic strokes (women aged 55-79 years).

[3]Pregnant women at 12-16 weeks gestation or at first prenatal visit, if later.

[4]Refer women whose family history is associated with an increased risk for deleterious mutations in BRCA1 or BRCA 2 genes for *genetic counseling and evaluation for BRCA testing.*

[5]Engage in shared, informed decisionmaking and offer to prescribe risk-reducing medications, if appropriate, to women aged ≥35 years without prior breast cancer diagnosis who are at increased risk.

[6]Biennial screening mammography for women aged 50 to 74 years. Note: The Department of Health and Human Services, in implementing the Affordable Care Act, follows the 2002 USPSTF recommendation for screening mammography, with or without clinical breast examination, every 1-2 years for women aged 40 and older.

[7]Interventions during pregnancy and after birth to promote and support breastfeeding.

[8]Screen with cytology every 3 years (women ages 21 to 65) or co-test (cytology/HPV testing) every 5 years (women ages 30-65).

[9]Sexually active women 24 and younger and other asymptomatic women at increased risk for infection. Asymptomatic pregnant women 24 and younger and others at increased risk.

[10]Adults aged 50-75 using fecal occult blood testing, sigmoidoscopy, or colonoscopy.

[11]Newborns.

[12]When staff-assisted depression care supports are in place to assure accurate diagnosis, effective treatment, and followup.

3

13 Asymptomatic adults with sustained blood pressure greater than 135/80 mg Hg.

14 Provide intervention (exercise or physical therapy and/or vitamin D supplementation) to community-dwelling adults ≥65 years at increased risk for falls.

15 All women planning or capable of pregnancy take a daily supplement containing 0.4 to 0.8 mg (400 to 800 μg) of folic acid.

16 Asymptomatic pregnant women after 24 weeks of gestation.

17 Newborns.

18 Sexually active women, including pregnant women 25 and younger, or at increased risk for infection.

19 Newborns.

20 Screen at first prenatal visit.

21 Persons at high risk for infection and adults born between 1945 and 1965.

22 All adolescents and adults ages 15 to 65 years and others who are at increased risk for HIV infection and all pregnant women.

23 Asymptomatic women of childbearing age; provide or refer women who screen positive to intervention services.

24 Routine iron supplementation for asymptomatic children aged 6 to 12 months who are at increased risk for iron deficiency anemia.

25 Routine screening in asymptomatic pregnant women.

26 Men aged 20-35 and women over age 20 who are at increased risk for coronary heart disease; all men aged 35 and older.

27 Asymptomatic adults aged 55 to 80 years who have a 30 pack-year smoking history and currently smoke or have quit smoking within the past 15 years.

28 Adolescents (age 12 to 18) when systems are in place to ensure accurate diagnosis, psychotherapy, and followup.

29 Patients with a body mass index of 30 kg/m2 or higher should be offered or referred to intensive, multicomponent behavioral interventions.

30 Screen children aged 6 years and older; offer or refer for intensive counseling and behavioral interventions.

31 Women aged 65 years and older and women under age 65 whose 10-year fracture risk is equal to or greater than that of a 65-year-old white woman without additional risk factors.

32 Newborns.

33 All sexually active adolescents and adults at increased risk for STIs.

34 Newborns.

35 Children, adolescents, and young adults aged 10 to 24 years.

36 Ask all adults about tobacco use and provide tobacco cessation interventions for those who use tobacco; provide augmented, pregnancy-tailored counseling for those pregnant women who smoke.

37 Provide interventions to prevent initiation of tobacco use in school-aged children and adolescents.

38 Screen children ages 3 to 5 years.

Clinical Summaries of Recommendations for Adults

All clinical summaries in this Guide are abridged recommendations. To see the full recommendation statements and recommendations published after March 2014, go to www.USPreventiveServicesTaskForce.org.

Abdominal Aortic Aneurysm

Title	Screening for Abdominal Aortic Aneurysm		
Population	Men ages 65 to 75 years who have ever smoked	Men ages 65 to 75 years who have never smoked	Women ages 65 to 75 years
Recommendation	**Screen once for abdominal aortic aneurysm with ultrasonography.** **Grade: B**	**No recommendation for or against screening.** **Grade: C**	**Do not screen for abdominal aortic aneurysm.** **Grade: D**

Risk Assessment	The major risk factors for abdominal aortic aneurysm include male sex, a history of ever smoking (defined as 100 cigarettes in a person's lifetime), and age of 65 years or older.
Screening Tests	Screening abdominal ultrasonography is an accurate test when performed in a setting with adequate quality assurance (i.e., in an accredited facility with credentialed technologists). Abdominal palpation has poor accuracy and is not an adequate screening test.
Timing of Screening	One-time screening to detect an abdominal aortic aneurysm using ultrasonography is sufficient. There is negligible health benefit in re-screening those who have normal aortic diameter on initial screening.
Interventions	Open surgical repair of an aneurysm of at least 5.5 cm leads to decreased abdominal aortic aneurysm-related mortality in the long term; however, there are major harms associated with this procedure.
Balance of Benefits and Harms	In men ages 65 to 75 years who have ever smoked, the benefits of screening for abdominal aortic aneurysm outweigh the harms.	In men ages 65 to 75 years who have never smoked, the balance between the benefits and harms of screening for abdominal aortic aneurysm is too close to make a general recommendation for this population.	The potential overall benefit of screening for abdominal aortic aneurysm among women ages 65 to 75 years is low because of the small number of abdominal aortic aneurysm-related deaths in this population and the harms associated with surgical repair.
Other Relevant USPSTF Recommendations	The USPSTF has made recommendations on screening for carotid artery stenosis, coronary heart disease, high blood pressure, lipid disorders, and peripheral arterial disease. These recommendations are available at http://www.uspreventiveservicestaskforce.org/.

For a summary of the evidence systematically reviewed in making this recommendation, the full recommendation statement, and supporting documents, please go to http://www.uspreventiveservicestaskforce.org/.

Alcohol Misuse

Title	Screening and Behavioral Counseling Interventions in Primary Care To Reduce Alcohol Misuse	
Population	Adults aged 18 years or older	Adolescents
Recommendation	**Screen for alcohol misuse and provide brief behavioral counseling interventions to persons engaged in risky or hazardous drinking.** **Grade: B**	No recommendation. Grade: I (Insufficient Evidence)

Screening Tests	Numerous screening instruments can detect alcohol misuse in adults with acceptable sensitivity and specificity. The USPSTF prefers the following tools for alcohol misuse screening in the primary care setting: 1. AUDIT 2. Abbreviated AUDIT-C 3. Single-question screening, such as asking, "How many times in the past year have you had 5 (for men) or 4 (for women and all adults older than 65 years) or more drinks in a day?"
Behavioral Counseling Interventions	Counseling interventions in the primary care setting can improve unhealthy alcohol consumption behaviors in adults engaging in risky or hazardous drinking. Behavioral counseling interventions for alcohol misuse vary in their specific components, administration, length, and number of interactions. Brief multicontact behavioral counseling seems to have the best evidence of effectiveness; very brief behavioral counseling has limited effect.
Balance of Benefits and Harms	There is a moderate net benefit to alcohol misuse screening and brief behavioral counseling interventions in the primary care setting for adults aged 18 years or older. The evidence on alcohol misuse screening and brief behavioral counseling interventions in the primary care setting for adolescents is insufficient, and the balance of benefits and harms cannot be determined.
Other Relevant USPSTF Recommendations	The USPSTF has made recommendations on screening for illicit drug use and counseling and interventions to prevent tobacco use. These recommendations are available at http://www.uspreventiveservicestaskforce.org/.

For a summary of the evidence systematically reviewed in making this recommendation, the full recommendation statement, and supporting documents, please go to http://www.uspreventiveservicestaskforce.org/.

Aspirin for the Prevention of Cardiovascular Disease

Title	Aspirin for the Prevention of Cardiovascular Disease			
Population	Men age 45-79 years	Women age 55-79 years	Men age <45 years	Women age <55 years	Men & Women age ≥80 years
Recommendation	Encourage aspirin use when potential CVD benefit (MIs prevented) outweighs potential harm of GI hemorrhage.	Encourage aspirin use when potential CVD benefit (strokes prevented) outweighs potential harm of GI hemorrhage.	Do not encourage aspirin use for MI prevention.	Do not encourage aspirin use for stroke prevention.	No Recommendation
	Grade: A		Grade: D		Grade: I (Insufficient Evidence)

How to Use This Recommendation	Shared decisionmaking is strongly encouraged with individuals whose risk is close to (either above or below) the estimates of 10-year risk levels indicated below. As the potential CVD benefit increases above harms, the recommendation to take aspirin should become stronger.
	To determine whether the potential benefit of MIs prevented (men) and strokes prevented (women) outweighs the potential harm of increased GI hemorrhage, both 10-year CVD risk and age must be considered.
	Risk level at which CVD events prevented (benefit) exceeds GI harms

Men 10-year CHD risk		Women 10-year stroke risk	
Age 45-59 years	≥4%	Age 55-59 years	≥3%
Age 60-69 years	≥9%	Age 60-69 years	≥8%
Age 70-79 years	≥12%	Age 70-79 years	≥11%

The table above applies to adults who are not taking NSAIDs and who do not have upper GI pain or a history of GI ulcers.

NSAID use and history of GI ulcers raise the risk of serious GI bleeding considerably and should be considered in determining the balance of benefits and harms. NSAID use combined with aspirin use approximately quadruples the risk of serious GI bleeding compared to the risk with aspirin use alone. The rate of serious bleeding in aspirin users is approximately 2-3 times higher in patients with a history of GI ulcers.

Risk Assessment	**For men:** Risk factors for CHD include age, diabetes, total cholesterol level, HDL level, blood pressure, and smoking. CHD risk estimation tool: cvdrisk.nhlbi.nih.gov/calculator.asp
	For women: Risk factors for ischemic stroke include age, high blood pressure, diabetes, smoking, history of CVD, atrial fibrillation, and left ventricular hypertrophy. Stroke risk estimation tool: http://www.westernstroke.org/index.php?header_name=stroke_tools.gif&main=stroke_tools.php

Other Relevant USPSTF Recommendations	The USPSTF has made recommendations on screening for abdominal aortic aneurysm, carotid artery stenosis, coronary heart disease, high blood pressure, lipid disorders, and peripheral arterial disease. These recommendations are available at http://www.uspreventiveservicestaskforce.org.

Abbreviations: CHD = coronary heart disease, CVD = cardiovascular disease, GI = gastrointestinal, HDL = high-density lipoprotein, MI = myocardial infarction, NSAIDs = nonsteroidal anti-inflammatory drugs.

For a summary of the evidence systematically reviewed in making these recommendations, the full recommendation statement, and supporting documents, please go to http://www.uspreventiveservicestaskforce.org.

Aspirin or NSAIDs for Prevention Of Colorectal Cancer

Title	Routine Aspirin or Nonsteroidal Anti-Inflammatory Drug (NSAID) Use for the Primary Prevention of Colorectal Cancer
Population	Asymptomatic adults at average risk for colorectal cancer
Recommendation	Do not use aspirin or NSAIDs for the prevention of colorectal cancer. Grade: D

Risk Assessment	The major risk factors for colorectal cancer are older age (older than age 50 years), family history (having two or more first- or second-degree relatives with colorectal cancer), and African American race.
Balance of Benefits and Harms	Aspirin and NSAIDs, taken in higher doses for longer periods, reduce the incidence of adenomatous polyps. However, there is poor evidence that aspirin and NSAID use leads to a reduction in colorectal cancer-associated mortality. Aspirin increases the incidence of gastrointestinal bleeding and hemorrhagic stroke; NSAIDs increase the incidence of gastrointestinal bleeding and renal impairment, especially in the elderly. The USPSTF concluded that the harms outweigh the benefits of aspirin and NSAID use for the prevention of colorectal cancer.
Other Relevant USPSTF Recommendations	The USPSTF has made recommendations on screening for colorectal cancer and aspirin use for the prevention of cardiovascular disease. These recommendations are available at http://www.uspreventiveservicestaskforce.org/.

For a summary of the evidence systematically reviewed in making this recommendation, the full recommendation statement, and supporting documents, please go to http://www.uspreventiveservicestaskforce.org/.

Bacterial Vaginosis in Pregnancy

Title	Screening for Bacterial Vaginosis in Pregnancy to Prevent Preterm Delivery	
Population	Asymptomatic pregnant women without risk factors for preterm delivery	Asymptomatic pregnant women with risk factors for preterm delivery
Recommendation	Do not screen. Grade: D	No recommendation. Grade: I (Insufficient Evidence)

Risk Assessment	Risk factors of preterm delivery include: ● African-American women. ● Pelvic infection. ● Previous preterm delivery. Bacterial vaginosis is more common among African-American women, women of low socioeconomic status, and women who have previously delivered low-birth-weight infants.
Screening Tests	Bacterial vaginosis is diagnosed using Amsel's clinical criteria or Gram stain. When using Amsel's criteria, 3 out of 4 criteria must be met to make a clinical diagnosis: 1. Vaginal pH >4.7. 2. The presence of clue cells on wet mount. 3. Thin homogeneous discharge. 4. Amine 'fishy odor' when potassium hydroxide is added to the discharge.
Screening Intervals	Not applicable.
Treatment	Treatment is appropriate for pregnant women with symptomatic bacterial vaginosis infection. Oral metronidazole and oral clindamycin, as well as vaginal metronidazole gel or clindamycin cream, are used to treat bacterial vaginosis. The optimal treatment regimen is unclear.[1]

[1]The Centers for Disease Control and Prevention (CDC) recommends 250 mg oral metronidazole 3 times a day for 7 days as the treatment for bacterial vaginosis in pregnancy.

For a summary of the evidence systematically reviewed in making these recommendations, the full recommendation statement, and supporting documents, please go to http://www.uspreventiveservicestaskforce.org.

Bacteriuria

Title	Screening for Asymptomatic Bacteriuria in Adults	
Population	All pregnant women	Men and nonpregnant women
Recommendation	Screen with urine culture. Grade: A	Do not screen. Grade: D

Detection and Screening Tests	Asymptomatic bacteriuria can be reliably detected through urine culture. The presence of at least 10^5 colony-forming units per mL of urine, of a single uropathogen, and in a midstream clean-catch specimen is considered a positive test result.	
Screening Intervals	A clean-catch urine specimen should be collected for screening culture at 12-16 weeks' gestation or at the first prenatal visit, if later. The optimal frequency of subsequent urine testing during pregnancy is uncertain.	Do not screen.
Benefits of Detection and Early Treatment	The detection and treatment of asymptomatic bacteriuria with antibiotics significantly reduces the incidence of symptomatic maternal urinary tract infections and low birthweight.	Screening men and nonpregnant women for asymptomatic bacteriuria is ineffective in improving clinical outcomes.
Harms of Detection and Early Treatment	Potential harms associated with treatment of asymptomatic bacteriuria include: • Adverse effects from antibiotics. • Development of bacterial resistance.	
Other Relevant USPSTF Recommendations	Additional USPSTF recommendations involving screening for infectious conditions during pregnancy can be found at www.uspreventiveservicestaskforce.org/recommendations.htm#obstetric and www.uspreventiveservicestaskforce.org/recommendations.htm#infectious.	

For a summary of the evidence systematically reviewed in making these recommendations, the full recommendation statement, and supporting documents, please go to http://www.uspreventiveservicestaskforce.org.

Bladder Cancer

Title	Screening for Bladder Cancer
Population	Asymptomatic adults
Recommendation	No recommendation. Grade: I (Insufficient Evidence)

Risk Assessment	Risk factors for bladder cancer include: ● Smoking ● Occupational exposure to carcinogens (e.g., rubber, chemical, and leather industries) ● Male sex ● Older age ● White race ● Infections caused by certain bladder parasites ● Family or personal history of bladder cancer
Screening Tests	Screening tests for bladder cancer include: ● Microscopic urinalysis for hematuria ● Urine cytology ● Urine biomarkers
Interventions	The principal treatment for superficial bladder cancer is transurethral resection of the bladder tumor, which may be combined with adjuvant radiation therapy, chemotherapy, biologic therapies, or photodynamic therapies. Radical cystectomy, often with adjuvant chemotherapy, is used in cases of surgically resectable invasive bladder cancer.
Balance of Benefits and Harms	There is inadequate evidence that treatment of screen-detected bladder cancer leads to improved morbidity or mortality. There is inadequate evidence on harms of screening for bladder cancer.
Suggestions for Practice	In deciding whether to screen for bladder cancer, clinicians should consider the following: ● *Potential preventable burden:* early detection of tumors with malignant potential could have an important impact on the mortality rate of bladder cancer. ● *Potential harms:* false-positive results may lead to anxiety and unneeded evaluations, diagnostic-related harms from cystoscopy and biopsy, harms from labeling and unnecessary treatments, and overdiagnosis. ● *Current practice:* screening tests used in primary practice include microscopic urinalysis for hematuria and urine cytology; urine biomarkers are not commonly used in part because of cost. Patients with positive findings are typically referred to a urologist for further evaluation.
Other Relevant USPSTF Recommendations	Recommendations on screening for other types of cancer can be found at www.uspreventiveservicestaskforce.org.

For a summary of the evidence systematically reviewed in making these recommendations, the full recommendation statement, and supporting documents, please go to http://www.uspreventiveservicestaskforce.org.

BRCA-Related Cancer in Women

Title	Risk Assessment, Genetic Counseling, and Genetic Testing for BRCA-Related Cancer In Women
Population	Asymptomatic women who have not been diagnosed with BRCA-related cancer
Recommendation	**Screen women whose family history may be associated with an increased risk for potentially harmful BRCA mutations. Women with positive screening results should receive genetic counseling and, if indicated after counseling, BRCA testing.** Grade: B	**Do not routinely recommend genetic counseling or BRCA testing to women whose family history is not associated with an increased risk for potentially harmful BRCA mutations.** Grade: D

Risk Assessment	Family history factors associated with increased likelihood of potentially harmful BRCA mutations include breast cancer diagnosis before age 50 years, bilateral breast cancer, family history of breast and ovarian cancer, presence of breast cancer in ≥1 male family member, multiple cases of breast cancer in the family, ≥1 or more family member with 2 primary types of BRCA-related cancer, and Ashkenazi Jewish ethnicity. Several familial risk stratification tools are available to determine the need for in-depth genetic counseling, such as the Ontario Family History Assessment Tool, Manchester Scoring System, Referral Screening Tool, Pedigree Assessment Tool, and FHS-7.	
Screening Tests	Genetic risk assessment and BRCA mutation testing are generally multistep processes involving identification of women who may be at increased risk for potentially harmful mutations, followed by genetic counseling by suitably trained health care providers and genetic testing of selected high-risk women when indicated. Tests for BRCA mutations are highly sensitive and specific for known mutations, but interpretation of results is complex and generally requires posttest counseling.	
Treatment	Interventions in women who are BRCA mutation carriers include earlier, more frequent, or intensive cancer screening; risk-reducing medications (e.g., tamoxifen or raloxifene); and risk-reducing surgery (e.g., mastectomy or salpingo-oophorectomy).	
Balance of Benefits and Harms	In women whose family history is associated with an increased risk for potentially harmful BRCA mutations, the net benefit of genetic testing and early intervention is moderate.	In women whose family history is not associated with an increased risk for potentially harmful BRCA mutations, the net benefit of genetic testing and early intervention ranges from minimal to potentially harmful.
Other Relevant USPSTF Recommendations	The USPSTF has made recommendations on medications for the reduction of breast cancer risk and screening for ovarian cancer. These recommendations are available at www.uspreventiveservicestaskforce.org.	

For a summary of the evidence systematically reviewed in making this recommendation, the full recommendation statement, and supporting documents, please go to www.uspreventiveservicestaskforce.org.

Breast Cancer (Preventive Medications)

Title	Medications for Risk Reduction of Primary Breast Cancer in Women
Population	Asymptomatic women aged ≥35 years without a prior diagnosis of breast cancer who are at increased risk for the disease	Asymptomatic women aged ≥35 years without a prior diagnosis of breast cancer who are not at increased risk for the disease
Recommendation	Engage in shared, informed decision making and offer to prescribe risk-reducing medications, if appropriate. **Grade: B**	Do not prescribe risk-reducing medications. **Grade: D**

Risk Assessment	Important risk factors for breast cancer include patient age, race/ethnicity, age at menarche, age at first live childbirth, personal history of ductal or lobular carcinoma in situ, number of first-degree relatives with breast cancer, personal history of breast biopsy, body mass index, menopause status or age, breast density, estrogen and progestin use, smoking, alcohol use, physical activity, and diet. Available risk assessment models can accurately predict the number of breast cancer cases that may arise in certain study populations, but their ability to accurately predict which women will develop breast cancer is modest.
Preventive Medications	The selective estrogen receptor modulators tamoxifen and raloxifene have been shown to reduce the incidence of invasive breast cancer in women who are at increased risk for the disease. Tamoxifen has been approved for this use in women age 35 years or older, and raloxifene has been approved for this use in postmenopausal women. The usual daily doses for tamoxifen and raloxifene are 20 mg and 60 mg, respectively, for 5 years.
Balance of Benefits and Harms	There is a moderate net benefit from use of tamoxifen and raloxifene to reduce the incidence of invasive breast cancer in women who are at increased risk for the disease.	The potential harms of tamoxifen and raloxifene outweigh the potential benefits for breast cancer risk reduction in women who are not at increased risk for the disease. Potential harms include thromboembolic events, endometrial cancer, and cataracts.
Other Relevant USPSTF Recommendations	The USPSTF has made recommendations on risk assessment, genetic counseling, and genetic testing for BRCA-related cancer, as well as screening for breast cancer. These recommendations are available at http://www.uspreventiveservicestaskforce.org/.

For a summary of the evidence systematically reviewed in making this recommendation, the full recommendation statement, and supporting documents, please go to http://www.uspreventiveservicestaskforce.org/.

Breast Cancer (Screening)

Title	Screening for Breast Cancer: Using Film Mammography		
Population	Women aged 40-49 years	Women aged 50-74 years	Women aged ≥75 years
Recommendation	Individualize decision to begin biennial screening according to the patient's circumstances and values. Grade: C	Screen every 2 years. Grade: B	No recommendation. Grade: I (Insufficient Evidence)

Risk Assessment	This recommendation applies to women aged ≥40 years who are not at increased risk by virtue of a known genetic mutation or history of chest radiation. Increasing age is the most important risk factor for most women.
Screening Tests	Standardization of film mammography has led to improved quality. Refer patients to facilities certified under the Mammography Quality Standards Act (MQSA), listed at http://www.accessdata.fda.gov/scripts/cdrh/cfdocs/cfMQSA/mqsa.cfm
Timing of Screening	Evidence indicates that biennial screening is optimal. A biennial schedule preserves most of the benefit of annual screening and cuts the harms nearly in half. A longer interval may reduce the benefit.
Balance of Benefits and Harms	There is convincing evidence that screening with film mammography reduces breast cancer mortality, with a greater absolute reduction for women aged 50 to 74 years than for younger women. Harms of screening include psychological harms, additional medical visits, imaging, and biopsies in women without cancer, inconvenience due to false-positive screening results, harms of unnecessary treatment, and radiation exposure. Harms seem moderate for each age group. False-positive results are a greater concern for younger women; treatment of cancer that would not become clinically apparent during a woman's life (overdiagnosis) is an increasing problem as women age.
Rationale for No Recommendation (I Statement)	Among women 75 years or older, evidence of benefit is lacking.
Other Relevant USPSTF Recommendations	USPSTF recommendations on screening for genetic susceptibility for breast cancer and chemoprevention of breast cancer are available at http://www.uspreventiveservicestaskforce.org.

The U.S. Department of Health and Human Services, in implementing the Affordable Care Act under the standard it sets out in revised Section 2713(a)(5) of the Public Health Service Act, utilizes the 2002 recommendation on breast cancer screening of the U.S. Preventive Services Task Force. For clinical summary of 2002 Recommendation, see Appendix F.

For a summary of the evidence systematically reviewed in making these recommendations, the full recommendation statement, and supporting documents, please go to

Breastfeeding

Title	Primary Care Interventions to Promote Breastfeeding		
Population	Pregnant women	New mothers	The mother's partner, other family members, and friends	Infants and young children
Recommendation	**Promote and support breastfeeding.** Grade: B		

Benefits of Breastfeeding	Mothers Less likelihood of breast and ovarian cancer	Infants Fewer ear infections, lower-respiratory-tract infections, and gastrointestinal infections	Young children Less likelihood of asthma, type 2 diabetes, and obesity
Interventions to Promote Breastfeeding	Interventions to promote and support breastfeeding have been found to increase the rates of initiation, duration, and exclusivity of breastfeeding. Consider multiple strategies, including: • Formal breastfeeding education for mothers and families • Direct support of mothers during breastfeeding • Training of primary care staff about breastfeeding and techniques for breastfeeding support • Peer support Interventions that include both prenatal and postnatal components may be most effective at increasing breastfeeding duration. In rare circumstances, for example for mothers with HIV and infants with galactosemia, breastfeeding is not recommended. Interventions to promote breastfeeding should empower individuals to make informed choices supported by the best available evidence.		
Implementation	System-level interventions with senior leadership support may be more likely to be sustained over time.		

For a summary of the evidence systematically reviewed in making these recommendations, the full recommendation statement, and supporting documents, please go to http://www.uspreventiveservicestaskforce.org.

Carotid Artery Stenosis

Title	Screening for Carotid Artery Stenosis
Population	Adult general population[1]
Recommendation	**Do not screen with ultrasound or other screening tests.** **Grade: D**

Risk Assessment	The major risk factors for carotid artery stenosis (CAS) include: older age, male gender, hypertension, smoking, hypercholesterolemia, and heart disease. However, accurate, reliable risk assessment tools are not available.
Balance of Benefits and Harms	Harms outweigh benefits. In the general population, screening with carotid duplex ultrasound would result in more false-positive results than true positive results. This would lead either to surgeries that are not indicated or to confirmatory angiography. As the result of these procedures, some people would suffer serious harms (death, stroke, and myocardial infarction) that outweigh the potential benefit surgical treatment may have in preventing stroke.
Other Relevant Recommendations from the USPSTF	Adults should be screened for hypertension, hyperlipidemia, and smoking. Clinicians should discuss aspirin chemoprevention with patients at increased risk for cardiovascular disease. These recommendations and related evidence are available at http://www.uspreventiveservicestaskforce.org.

[1]This recommendation applies to adults without neurological symptoms and without a history of transient ischemic attacks (TIA) or stroke. If otherwise eligible, an individual who has a carotid area TIA should be evaluated promptly for consideration of carotid endarterectomy.

For a summary of the evidence systematically reviewed in making these recommendations, the full recommendation statement, and supporting documents, please go to http://www.uspreventiveservicestaskforce.org.

Cervical Cancer

Title	Screening for Cervical Cancer				
Population	Women ages 21 to 65	Women ages 30 to 65	Women younger than age 21	Women older than age 65 who have had adequate prior screening and are not high risk	Women after hysterectomy with removal of the cervix and with no history of high-grade precancer or cervical cancer	Women younger than age 30
Recommendation	Screen with cytology (Pap smear) every 3 years. Grade: A	Screen with cytology every 3 years or co-testing (cytology/HPV testing) every 5 years Grade: A	Do not screen. Grade: D	Do not screen. Grade: D	Do not screen. Grade: D	Do not screen with HPV testing (alone or with cytology) Grade: D

Risk Assessment	Human papillomavirus (HPV) infection is associated with nearly all cases of cervical cancer. Other factors that put a woman at increased risk of cervical cancer include HIV infection, a compromised immune system, in utero exposure to diethylstilbestrol, and previous treatment of a high-grade precancerous lesion or cervical cancer.
Screening Tests and Interval	Screening women ages 21 to 65 every 3 years with cytology provides a reasonable balance between benefits and harms. Screening with cytology more often than every 3 years confers little additional benefit, with large increases in harms. HPV testing combined with cytology (co-testing) every 5 years in women ages 30 to 65 years offers a comparable balance of benefits and harms, and is therefore a reasonable alternative for women in this age group who would prefer to extend the screening interval.
Timing of Screening	Screening earlier than age 21 years, regardless of sexual history, leads to more harms than benefits. Clinicians and patients should base the decision to end screening on whether the patient meets the criteria for adequate prior testing and appropriate follow-up, per established guidelines.
Interventions	Screening aims to identify high-grade precancerous cervical lesions to prevent development of cervical cancer and early-stage asymptomatic invasive cervical cancer. High-grade lesions may be treated with ablative and excisional therapies, including cryotherapy, laser ablation, loop excision, and cold knife conization. Early-stage cervical cancer may be treated with surgery (hysterectomy) or chemoradiation.
Balance of Benefits and Harms	The benefits of screening with cytology every 3 years substantially outweigh the harms.	The benefits of screening with co-testing (cytology/HPV testing) every 5 years outweigh the harms.	The harms of screening earlier than age 21 years outweigh the benefits.	The benefits of screening after age 65 years do not outweigh the potential harms.	The harms of screening after hysterectomy outweigh the benefits.	The potential harms of screening with HPV testing (alone or with cytology) outweigh the potential benefits.
Other Relevant USPSTF Recommendations	The USPSTF has made recommendations on screening for breast cancer and ovarian cancer, as well as genetic risk assessment and *BRCA* mutation testing for breast and ovarian cancer susceptibility. These recommendations are available at http://www.uspreventiveservicestaskforce.org/.

For a summary of the evidence systematically reviewed in making this recommendation, the full recommendation statement, and supporting documents, please go to http://www.uspreventiveservicestaskforce.org/.

Chlamydial Infection

Title	Screening for Chlamydial Infection						
	Non-pregnant women			Pregnant women			Men
	24 years and younger	25 years and older		24 years and younger	25 years and older		
Population	Includes adolescents	Not at increased risk	At increased risk	Includes adolescents	Not at increased risk	At increased risk	
Recommendation	Screen if sexually active. Grade: A	Do not automatically screen. Grade: C	Screen. Grade: A	Screen. Grade: B	Do not automatically screen. Grade: C	Screen. Grade: B	No recommendation. Grade: I (Insufficient Evidence[1])

Risk Assessment	**Age:** Women and men aged 24 years and younger are at greatest risk. **History of:** previous chlamydial infection or other sexually transmitted infections, new or multiple sexual partners, inconsistent condom use, sex work. **Demographics:** African-Americans and Hispanic women and men have higher prevalence rates than the general population in many communities.
Screening Tests	Nucleic acid amplification tests (NAATs) can identify chlamydial infection in asymptomatic women (non-pregnant and pregnant) and asymptomatic men. NAATs have high specificity and sensitivity and can be used with urine and vaginal swabs.
Screening Intervals	**Non-Pregnant Women** The optimal interval for screening is not known. The CDC recommends that women at increased risk be screened at least annually.[2] **Pregnant Women** For women 24 years and younger and older women at increased risk: Screen at the first prenatal visit. For patients at continuing risk, or who are newly at risk: Screen in the 3rd trimester.
Treatment	The Centers for Disease Control and Prevention has outlined appropriate treatment at: http://www.cdc.gov/STD/treatment. Test and/or treat partners of patients treated for chlamydial infection.

[1]Chlamydial infection results in few sequelae in men. Therefore, the major benefit of screening men would be to reduce the likelihood that infected and untreated men would pass the infection to sexual partners. There is no evidence that screening men reduces the long-term consequences of chlamydial infection in women. Because of this lack of evidence, the USPSTF was not able to assess the balance of benefits and harms, and concluded that the evidence is insufficient to recommend for or against routinely screening men.

[2]Centers for Disease Control and Prevention. Sexually transmitted diseases treatment guidelines, 2006. *MMWR* 2006. 55(No. RR-11).

For a summary of the evidence systematically reviewed in making these recommendations, the full recommendation statement, and supporting documents, please go to http://www.uspreventiveservicestaskforce.org.

Chronic Kidney Disease

Title	Screening for Chronic Kidney Disease
Population	Asymptomatic adults without diagnosed chronic kidney disease (CKD)
Recommendation	No recommendation. Grade: I (Insufficient Evidence)

Risk Assessment	There is no generally accepted risk assessment tool for CKD or risk for complications of CKD. Diabetes and hypertension are well-established risk factors with strong links to CKD. Other risk factors for CKD include older age, cardiovascular disease, obesity, and family history.
Screening Tests	While there is insufficient evidence to recommend routine screening, the tests often suggested for screening that are feasible in primary care include testing the urine for protein (microalbuminuria or macroalbuminuria) and testing the blood for serum creatinine to estimate glomerular filtration rate.
Balance of Benefits and Harms	The USPSTF could not determine the balance between the benefits and harms of screening for CKD in asymptomatic adults.
Other Relevant USPSTF Recommendations	The USPSTF has made recommendations on screening for diabetes, hypertension, and obesity, as well as aspirin use for the prevention of cardiovascular disease. These recommendations are available at http://www.uspreventiveservicestaskforce.org/.

For a summary of the evidence systematically reviewed in making this recommendation, the full recommendation statement, and supporting documents, please go to http://www.uspreventiveservicestaskforce.org/.

21

Chronic Obstructive Pulmonary Disease

Title	Screening for Chronic Obstructive Pulmonary Disease Using Spirometry
Population	Adult general population
Recommendation	**Do not screen for chronic obstructive pulmonary disease using spirometry.** **Grade: D**

Additional Population Information	This screening recommendation applies to healthy adults who do not recognize or report respiratory symptoms to a clinician. It does not apply to individuals with a family history of alpha-1 antitrypsin deficiency.
Risk Assessment	Risk factors for COPD include: • Current or past tobacco use. • Exposure to occupational and environmental pollutants. • Age 40 or older.
Screening Tests[1]	Spirometry can be performed in a primary care physician's office or a pulmonary testing laboratory. The USPSTF did not review evidence comparing the accuracy of spirometry performed in primary care versus referral settings. For individuals who present to clinicians complaining of chronic cough, increased sputum production, wheezing, or dyspnea, spirometry would be indicated as a diagnostic test for COPD, asthma, and other pulmonary diseases.
Other Approaches to the Prevention of Pulmonary Illnesses	These services should be offered to patients regardless of COPD status: • All current smokers should receive smoking cessation counseling and be offered pharmacologic therapies demonstrated to increase cessation rates. • All patients 50 years of age or older should be offered **influenza immunization** annually. • All patients 65 years of age or older should be offered one-time **pneumococcal immunization.**
Other Relevant USPSTF Recommendations	Clinicians should screen all adults for tobacco use and provide tobacco cessation interventions for those who use tobacco products. The USPSTF tobacco cessation counseling recommendation and supporting evidence are available at http://www.uspreventiveservicestaskforce.org/uspstf/uspstbac.htm.

[1]The potential benefit of spirometry-based screening for COPD is prevention of one or more exacerbations by treating patients found to have an airflow obstruction previously undetected. However, even in groups with the greatest prevalence of airflow obstruction, hundreds of patients would need to be screened with spirometry to defer one exacerbation.

For a summary of the evidence systematically reviewed in making these recommendations, the full recommendation statement, and supporting documents, please go to http://www.uspreventiveservicestaskforce.org.

Cognitive Impairment

Title	**Screening for Cognitive Impairment in Older Adults**
Population	Community-dwelling adults who are older than age 65 years and have no signs or symptoms of cognitive impairment
Recommendation	No recommendation. **Grade: I statement**

Risk Assessment	Increasing age is the strongest known risk factor for cognitive impairment. Other reported risk factors for cognitive impairment include cardiovascular risk factors (such as diabetes, tobacco use, hypercholesterolemia, and hypertension), head trauma, learning disabilities (such as Down syndrome), depression, alcohol abuse, physical frailty, low education level, low social support, and having never been married.
Screening Tests	Screening tests for cognitive impairment in the clinical setting generally include asking patients to perform a series of tasks that assess 1 or more cognitive domains (memory, attention, language, and visuospatial or executive functioning). The most widely studied instrument is the Mini-Mental State Examination. Other instruments with more limited evidence include the Clock Draw Test, Mini-Cog, Memory Impairment Screen, Abbreviated Mental Test, Short Portable Mental Status Questionnaire, Free and Cued Selective Reminding Test, 7-Minute Screen, Telephone Interview for Cognitive Status, and Informant Questionnaire on Cognitive Decline in the Elderly.
Treatment	Pharmacologic treatments approved by the U.S. Food and Drug Administration include acetylcholinesterase inhibitors and memantine. Nonpharmacologic interventions include cognitive training, lifestyle behavioral interventions, exercise, educational interventions, and multidisciplinary care interventions. Some interventions focus on the caregiver and aim to improve caregiver morbidity and delay institutionalization of persons with dementia.
Balance of Benefits and Harms	The evidence on screening for cognitive impairment is lacking, and the balance of benefits and harms cannot be determined.
Other Relevant USPSTF Recommendations	The USPSTF has made recommendations related to several of the risk factors for cognitive impairment, including counseling on tobacco cessation, alcohol use, healthful diet, physical activity, and falls prevention and screening for high cholesterol, hypertension, and depression. These recommendations are available at http://www.uspreventiveservicestaskforce.org/.

For a summary of the evidence systematically reviewed in making this recommendation, the full recommendation statement, and supporting documents, please go to http://www.uspreventiveservicestaskforce.org/.

Colorectal Cancer

Title	Screening for Colorectal Cancer		
Population[1]	Adults age 50 to 75 years	Adults age 76 to 85 years	Adults older than 85
Recommendation	Screen with high sensitivity fecal occult blood testing (FOBT), sigmoidoscopy, or colonoscopy. Grade: A	Do not automatically screen. Grade: C	Do not screen. Grade: D
	For all populations, evidence is insufficient to assess the benefits and harms of screening with computerized tomography colonography (CTC) and fecal DNA testing. Grade: I (Insufficient Evidence)		

Screening Tests	High sensitivity FOBT, sigmoidoscopy with FOBT, and colonoscopy are effective in decreasing colorectal cancer mortality. The risks and benefits of these screening methods vary. Colonoscopy and flexible sigmoidoscopy (to a lesser degree) entail possible serious complications.
Screening Test Intervals	Intervals for recommended screening strategies: • Annual screening with high-sensitivity fecal occult blood testing • Sigmoidoscopy every 5 years, with high-sensitivity fecal occult blood testing every 3 years • Screening colonoscopy every 10 years
Balance of Benefits and Harms	The benefits of screening outweigh the potential harms for 50- to 75-year-olds.	The likelihood that detection and early intervention will yield a mortality benefit declines after age 75 because of the long average time between adenoma development and cancer diagnosis.
Implementation	Focus on strategies that maximize the number of individuals who get screened. Practice shared decisionmaking; discussions with patients should incorporate information on test quality and availability. Individuals with a personal history of cancer or adenomatous polyps are followed by a surveillance regimen, and screening guidelines are not applicable.
Other Relevant USPSTF Recommendations	The USPSTF recommends against the use of aspirin or nonsteroidal anti-inflammatory drugs for the primary prevention of colorectal cancer. This recommendation is available at http://www.uspreventiveservicestaskforce.org.

[1]These recommendations do not apply to individuals with specific inherited syndromes (Lynch Syndrome or Familial Adenomatous Polyposis) or those with inflammatory bowel disease.

For a summary of the evidence systematically reviewed in making these recommendations, the full recommendation statement, and supporting documents, please go to http://www.uspreventiveservicestaskforce.org.

Coronary Heart Disease (Risk Assessment, Nontraditional Risk Factors)

Title	Using Nontraditional Risk Factors In Coronary Heart Disease Risk Assessment
Population	Asymptomatic men and women with no history of coronary heart disease (CHD), diabetes, or any CHD risk equivalent
Recommendation	No recommendation. Grade: I (Insufficient Evidence)

Risk Assessment	This recommendation applies to adult men and women classified at intermediate 10-year risk for CHD (10% to 20%) by traditional risk factors.
Importance	Coronary heart disease (CHD) is the most common cause of death in adults in the United States. Treatment to prevent CHD events by modifying risk factors is currently based on the Framingham risk model. If the classification of individuals at intermediate risk could be improved by using additional risk factors, treatment to prevent CHD might be targeted more effectively. Risk factors not currently part of the Framingham model (nontraditional risk factors) include high sensitivity C-reactive protein (hs-CRP), ankle-brachial index (ABI), leukocyte count, fasting blood glucose level, periodontal disease, carotid intima-media thickness, electron beam computed tomography, homocysteine level, and lipoprotein(a) level.
Balacne of Benefits and Harms	There is insufficient evidence to determine the percentage of intermediate-risk individuals who would be reclassified by screening with nontraditional risk factors, other than hs-CRP and ABI. For individuals reclassified as high-risk on the basis of hs-CRP or ABI scores, data are not available to determine whether they benefit from additional treatments. Little evidence is available to determine the harms of using nontraditional risk factors in screening. Potential harms include lifelong use of medications without proven benefit and psychological and other harms from being misclassified in a higher risk category.
Suggestions for practice	Clinicians should continue to use the Framingham model to assess CHD risk and guide risk-based preventive therapy. Adding nontraditional risk factors to CHD assessment would require additional patient and clinical staff time and effort. Routinely screening with nontraditional risk factors could result in lost opportunities to provide other important health services of proven benefit.
Other Relevant USPSTF Recommendations	USPSTF recommendations on risk assessment for CHD, the use of aspirin to prevent cardiovascular disease, and screening for high blood pressure can be accessed at http://www.uspreventiveservicestaskforce.org.

For a summary of the evidence systematically reviewed in making these recommendations, the full recommendation statement, and supporting documents, please go to http://www.uspreventiveservicestaskforce.org.

Coronary Heart Disease (Electrocardiography)

Title	Screening for Coronary Heart Disease with Electrocardiography	
Population	Asymptomatic adults at low risk for coronary heart disease (CHD) events	Asymptomatic adults at intermediate or high risk for CHD events
Recommendation	**Do not screen with resting or exercise electrocardiography (ECG).** **Grade: D**	**No recommendation.** **Grade: I (Insufficient Evidence)**

Risk Assessment	Several factors are associated with a higher risk for CHD events, including older age, male sex, high blood pressure, smoking, abnormal lipid levels, diabetes, obesity, and sedentary lifestyle. Calculators are available to ascertain a person's 10-year risk for a CHD event. Persons with a 10-year risk >20% are considered to be high-risk, those with a 10-year risk <10% are considered to be low-risk, and those in the 10%–20% range are considered to be intermediate-risk.
Screening Tests	Several abnormalities on resting and exercise ECG are associated with an increased risk for a serious CHD event. However, the incremental information offered by screening asymptomatic adults at low risk for a CHD event with resting or exercise ECG (beyond that obtained with conventional CHD risk factors) is highly unlikely to result in changes in risk stratification that would prompt interventions and ultimately reduce CHD-related events.
Balance of Benefits and Harms	The potential harms of screening for CHD with exercise or resting ECG equal or exceed the potential benefits in this population.	The USPSTF could not determine the balance between the benefits and harms of screening for CHD with resting or exercise ECG in this population.
Other Relevant USPSTF Recommendations	The USPSTF has made recommendations on screening for carotid artery stenosis, high blood pressure, lipid disorders, peripheral arterial disease, and obesity. These recommendations are available at http://www.uspreventiveservicestaskforce.org/.	

For a summary of the evidence systematically reviewed in making this recommendation, the full recommendation statement, and supporting documents, please go to http://www.uspreventiveservicestaskforce.org/.

Depression in Adults

Title	Screening for Depression in Adults
Population	Nonpregnant adults 18 years or older
Recommendation	Screen when staff-assisted depression care supports[1] are in place to assure accurate diagnosis, effective treatment, and followup. **Grade: B**	Do not automatically screen when staff-assisted depression care supports[1] are not in place. **Grade: C**
Risk Assessment	Persons at increased risk for depression are considered at risk throughout their lifetime. Groups at increased risk include persons with other psychiatric disorders, including substance misuse; persons with a family history of depression; persons with chronic medical diseases; and persons who are unemployed or of lower socioeconomic status. Also, women are at increased risk compared with men. However, the presence of risk factors alone cannot distinguish depressed patients from nondepressed patients.	
Screening Tests	Simple screening questions may perform as well as more complex instruments. Any positive screening test result should trigger a full diagnostic interview using standard diagnostic criteria.	
Timing of Screening	The optimal interval for screening is unknown. In older adults, significant depressive symptoms are associated with common life events, including medical illness, cognitive decline, bereavement, and institutional placement in residential or inpatient settings.	
Balance of Benefits and Harms		Limited evidence suggests that screening for depression in the absence of staff-assisted depression care does not improve depression outcomes.
Suggestions for Practice	"Staff-assisted depression care supports" refers to clinical staff that assists the primary care clinician by providing some direct depression care and/or coordination, case management, or mental health treatment.	
Relevant USPSTF Recommendations	Related USPSTF recommendations on screening for suicidality and screening children and adolescents for depression are available at http://www.uspreventiveservicestaskforce.org.	

[1]Go to the Suggestions for Practice section of this figure for further explanation.

For a summary of the evidence systematically reviewed in making these recommendations, the full recommendation statement, and supporting documents, please go to http://www.uspreventiveservicestaskforce.org.

Diabetes Mellitus

Title	Screening for Type 2 Diabetes Mellitus in Adults	
Population	Asymptomatic adults with sustained blood pressure greater than 135/80 mm Hg	Asymptomatic adults with sustained blood pressure 135/80 mm Hg or lower
Recommendation	Screen for type 2 diabetes mellitus. Grade: B	No recommendation. Grade: I (Insufficient Evidence)

Risk Assessment	These recommendations apply to adults with no symptoms of type 2 diabetes mellitus or evidence of possible complications of diabetes. Blood pressure measurement is an important predictor of cardiovascular complications in people with type 2 diabetes mellitus. The first step in applying this recommendation should be measurement of blood pressure (BP). Adults with treated or untreated BP >135/80 mm Hg should be screened for diabetes.
Screening Tests	Three tests have been used to screen for diabetes: ● Fasting plasma glucose (FPG). ● 2-hour postload plasma. ● Hemoglobin A1c. The American Diabetes Association (ADA) recommends screening with FPG, defines diabetes as FPG ≥ 126 mg/dL, and recommends confirmation with a repeated screening test on a separate day.
Screening Intervals	The optimal screening interval is not known. The ADA, on the basis of expert opinion, recommends an interval of every 3 years.
Suggestions for practice regarding insufficient evidence	When BP is ≤ 135/80 mm Hg, screening may be considered on an individual basis when knowledge of diabetes status would help inform decisions about coronary heart disease (CHD) preventive strategies, including consideration of lipid-lowering agents or aspirin. To determine whether screening would be helpful on an individual basis, information about 10-year CHD risk must be considered. For example, if CHD risk without diabetes was 17% and risk with diabetes was >20%, screening for diabetes would be helpful because diabetes status would determine lipid treatment. In contrast, if risk without diabetes was 10% and risk with diabetes was 15%, screening would not affect the decision to use lipid-lowering treatment.
Other relevant information from the USPSTF and the Community Preventive Services Task Force	Evidence and USPSTF recommendations regarding blood pressure, diet, physical activity, and obesity are available at http://www.uspreventiveservicestaskforce.org. The reviews and recommendations of the Community Preventive Services Task Force may be found at http://www.thecommunityguide.org.

For a summary of the evidence systematically reviewed in making these recommendations, the full recommendation statement, and supporting documents, please go to http://www.uspreventiveservicestaskforce.org.

Falls in Older Adults

Title	Prevention of Falls in Community-Dwelling Older Adults
Population	Community-dwelling adults aged 65 years and older who are at increased risk for falls	Community-dwelling adults aged 65 years and older
Recommendation	**Provide intervention consisting of exercise or physical therapy and/or vitamin D supplementation to prevent falls.** Grade: B	**Do not automatically perform an in-depth multifactorial risk assessment with comprehensive management of identified risks to prevent falls.** Grade: C

Risk Assessment	Primary care clinicians can consider the following factors to identify older adults at increased risk for falls: a history of falls, a history of mobility problems, and poor performance on the timed Get-Up-and-Go test.
Interventions	Effective exercise and physical therapy interventions include group classes and at-home physiotherapy strategies and range in intensity from very low (≤9 hours) to high (>75 hours). Benefit from vitamin D supplementation occurs by 12 months; the efficacy of treatment of shorter duration is unknown. The recommended daily allowance for vitamin D is 600 IU for adults aged 51 to 70 years and 800 IU for adults older than 70 years. Comprehensive multifactorial assessment and management interventions include assessment of multiple risk factors for falls and providing medical and social care to address factors identified during the assessment. In determining whether this service is appropriate in individual cases, patients and clinicians should consider the balance of benefits and harms on the basis of the circumstances of prior falls, medical comorbid conditions, and patient values.
Balance of Benefits and Harms	Exercise or physical therapy and vitamin D supplementation have a moderate benefit in preventing falls in older adults. Multifactorial risk assessment with comprehensive management of identified risks has at least a small benefit in preventing falls in older adults.
Other Relevant USPSTF Recommendations	The USPSTF has made recommendations on screening for osteoporosis. These recommendations are available at http://www.uspreventiveservicestaskforce.org/.

For a summary of the evidence systematically reviewed in making this recommendation, the full recommendation statement, and supporting documents, please go to http://www.uspreventiveservicestaskforce.org/.

29

Folic Acid Supplementation

Title	**Folic Acid for the Prevention of Neural Tube Defects**
Population	Women planning a pregnancy or capable of becoming pregnant
Recommendation	**Take a daily vitamin supplement containing 0.4 to 0.8 mg (400 to 800 μg) of folic acid.** **Grade: A**

Risk Assessment	Risk factors include: • A personal or family history of a pregnancy affected by a neural tube defect • The use of certain antiseizure medications • Mutations in folate-related enzymes • Maternal diabetes • Maternal obesity **Note:** This recommendation does not apply to women who have had a previous pregnancy affected by neural tube defects or women taking certain antiseizure medicines. These women may be advised to take higher doses of folic acid.
Timing of Medication	Start supplementation at least 1 month before conception. Continue through first 2 to 3 months of pregnancy.
Recommendations of Others	ACOG, AAFP, and most other organizations recommend 4 mg/d for women with a history of a pregnancy affected by a neural tube defect.

Abbreviations: AAFP = American Academy of Family Physicians; ACOG = American College of Obstetricians and Gynecologists.

For a summary of the evidence systematically reviewed in making these recommendations, the full recommendation statement, and supporting documents, please go to http://www.uspreventiveservicestaskforce.org.

Genital Herpes

Time	Screening for Genital Herpes	
Population	Asymptomatic pregnant women	Asymptomatic adolescents and adults
Recommendation	Do not screen for herpes simplex virus. Grade: D	Do not screen for herpes simplex virus. Grade: D
Screening Tests	Methods for detecting herpes simplex virus include viral culture, polymerase chain reaction, and antibody-based tests, such as the western blot assay and type-specific glycoprotein G serological tests.	
Interventions	There is limited evidence that the use of antiviral therapy in women with a history of recurrent infection, or performance of cesarean delivery in women with active herpes lesions at the time of delivery, decreases neonatal herpes infection. There is also limited evidence of the safety of antiviral therapy in pregnant women and neonates.	Antiviral therapy improves health outcomes in symptomatic persons (e.g., those with multiple recurrences); however, there is no evidence that the use of antiviral therapy improves health outcomes in those with asymptomatic infection. There are multiple efficacious regimens that may be used to prevent the recurrence of clinical genital herpes.
Balance of Benefits and Harms	The potential harms of screening asymptomatic pregnant women include false-positive test results, labeling, and anxiety, as well as false-negative tests and false reassurance, although these potential harms are not well studied. The USPSTF determined that there are no benefits associated with screening, and therefore the potential harms outweigh the benefits.	The potential harms of screening asymptomatic adolescents and adults include false-positive test results, labeling, and anxiety, although these potential harms are not well studied. The USPSTF determined the benefits of screening are minimal, at best, and the potential harms outweigh the potential benefits.
Other Relevant USPSTF Recommendations	The USPSTF has made recommendations on screening for chlamydia, gonorrhea, HIV, and several other sexually transmitted infections. These recommendations are available at http://www.uspreventiveservicestaskforce.org/.	

For a summary of the evidence systematically reviewed in making this recommendation, the full recommendation statement, and supporting documents, please go to http://www.uspreventiveservicestaskforce.org/.

Gestational Diabetes Mellitus

Title	Screening for Gestational Diabetes Mellitus	
Population	Asymptomatic pregnant women after 24 weeks of gestation	Asymptomatic pregnant women before 24 weeks of gestation
Recommendation	Screen for gestational diabetes mellitus (GDM). Grade: B	No recommendation. Grade: I (Insufficient Evidence)
Risk Assessment	Risk factors that increase a woman's risk for developing GDM include obesity, increased maternal age, history of GDM, family history of diabetes, and belonging to an ethnic group with increased risk of developing type 2 diabetes mellitus (Hispanic, Native American, South or East Asian, African American, or Pacific Islands descent).	
Screening Tests	There are 2 strategies used to screen for gestational diabetes in the United States. In the 2-step approach, the 50-g oral glucose challenge test is administered between 24 and 28 weeks of gestation in a nonfasting state. If the screening threshold is met or exceeded (7.22 mmol/L [130 mg/dL], 7.50 mmol/L [135 mg/dL], or 7.77 mmol/L [140 mg/dL]), patients receive the oral glucose tolerance test. A diagnosis of GDM is made when 2 or more glucose levels meet or exceed the specified glucose thresholds. In the 1-step approach, a 75-g glucose load is administered after fasting and plasma glucose levels are evaluated after 1 and 2 hours. GDM is diagnosed if 1 glucose value falls at or above the specified glucose threshold. Other methods of screening include fasting plasma glucose and screening based on risk factors. However, there is limited evidence on these alternative screening approaches.	
Treatment	Initial treatment includes moderate physical activity, dietary changes, support from diabetes educators and nutritionists, and glucose monitoring. If the patient's glucose is not controlled after these initial interventions, she may be prescribed medication (either insulin or oral hypoglycemic agents), undergo increased surveillance in prenatal care, and have changes in delivery management.	
Balance of Benefits and Harms	There is a moderate net benefit to screening for GDM after 24 weeks of gestation to reduce maternal and fetal complications.	The evidence for screening for GDM before 24 weeks of gestation is insufficient, and the balance of benefits and harms of screening cannot be determined.
Other Relevant USPSTF Recommendations	The USPSTF has made recommendations on screening for type 2 diabetes. These recommendations are available at http://www.uspreventiveservicestaskforce.org/.	

For a summary of the evidence systematically reviewed in making this recommendation, the full recommendation statement, and supporting documents, please go to http://www.uspreventiveservicestaskforce.org/.

Glaucoma

Title	Screening for Glaucoma
Population	Adults without vision symptoms who are seen in primary care
Recommendation	No recommendation. Grade: I (Insufficient Evidence)

Risk Assessment	Important risk factors for open-angle glaucoma are increased intraocular pressure, older age, family history of glaucoma, and African American race.
Screening Tests	Diagnosis of glaucoma is usually made on the basis of several tests that, when combined, evaluate the biologic structure and function of the optic nerve and intraocular pressure. Most tests that are available in a primary care setting do not have acceptable accuracy to detect glaucoma.
Treatment	The immediate physiologic goal and measure of effect of primary treatment of glaucoma is reduction in intraocular pressure. Treatments that are effective in reducing intraocular pressure include medications, laser therapy, and surgery. However, these treatments have potential harms, and their effectiveness in reducing patient-perceived impairment in vision-related function is uncertain.
Balance of Benefits and Harms	Evidence on the accuracy of screening tests, especially in primary care settings, and the benefits of screening or treatment to delay or prevent visual impairment or improve quality of life is inadequate. Therefore, the overall certainty of the evidence is low, and the USPSTF is unable to determine the balance of benefits and harms of screening for glaucoma in asymptomatic adults.
Other Relevant USPSTF Recommendations	The USPSTF has made recommendations on screening for impaired visual acuity in older adults. These recommendations are available at http://www.uspreventiveservicestaskforce.org/.

For a summary of the evidence systematically reviewed in making this recommendation, the full recommendation statement, and supporting documents, please go to http://www.uspreventiveservicestaskforce.org/.

Gonorrhea

Title	Screening for Gonorrhea			
Population	Sexually active women, including those who are pregnant, who are at increased risk for infection	Men who are at increased risk for infection	Men and women who are at low risk for infection	Pregnant women who are not at increased risk for infection
Recommendation	Screen for gonorrhea. Grade: B	No recommendation. Grade: I (Insufficient Evidence)	Do not screen for gonorrhea. Grade: D	No recommendation. Grade: I (Insufficient Evidence)
Risk Assessment	Women and men younger than age 25 years—including sexually active adolescents—are at highest risk for gonorrhea infection. Risk factors for gonorrhea include a history of previous gonorrhea infection, other sexually transmitted infections, new or multiple sexual partners, inconsistent condom use, sex work, and drug use. Risk factors for pregnant women are the same as for non-pregnant women.			
Screening Tests	Vaginal culture is an accurate screening test when transport conditions are suitable. Newer screening tests, including nucleic acid amplification and hybridization tests, have demonstrated improved sensitivity and comparable specificity when compared with cervical culture. Some newer tests can be used with urine and vaginal swabs, which enables screening when a pelvic examination is not performed.			
Timing of Screening	Screening is recommended at the first prenatal visit for pregnant women who are in a high-risk group for gonorrhea infection. For pregnant women who are at continued risk, and for those who acquire a new risk factor, a second screening should be conducted during the third trimester. The optimal interval for screening in the non-pregnant population is not known.			
Interventions	Genital gonorrhea infection in men and women, including pregnant women, may be treated with a third-generation cephalosporin. Because of increased prevalence of resistant organisms, fluoroquinolones should not be used to treat gonorrhea. Current guidelines for treating gonorrhea infection are available from the Centers for Disease Control and Prevention (http://www.cdc.gov/std/treatment).			
Balance of Benefits and Harms	The USPSTF concluded that the benefits of screening women at increased risk for gonorrhea infection outweigh the potential harms.	The USPSTF could not determine the balance of benefits and harms of screening for gonorrhea in men at increased risk for infection.	Given the low prevalence of gonorrhea infection in the general population, the USPSTF concluded that the potential harms of screening in low-prevalence populations outweigh the benefits.	The USPSTF could not determine the balance between the benefits and harms of screening for gonorrhea in pregnant women who are not at increased risk for infection.
Other Relevant USPSTF Recommendations	The USPSTF has also made a recommendation on ocular prophylaxis in newborns for gonococcal ophthalmia neonatorum. This recommendation is available at http://www.uspreventiveservicestaskforce.org/.			

For a summary of the evidence systematically reviewed in making this recommendation, the full recommendation statement, and supporting documents, please go to http://www.uspreventiveservicestaskforce.org/.

Healthful Diet and Physical Activity

Title	Behavioral Counseling Interventions to Promote A Healthful Diet and Physical Activity for Cardiovascular Disease Prevention in Adults
Population	General adult population without a known diagnosis of hypertension, diabetes, hyperlipidemia, or cardiovascular disease
Recommendation	**Although the correlation among healthful diet, physical activity, and the incidence of cardiovascular disease is strong, existing evidence indicates that the health benefit of initiating behavioral counseling in the primary care setting to promote a healthful diet and physical activity is small. Clinicians may choose to selectively counsel patients rather than incorporate counseling into the care of all adults in the general population.** Considerations: Issues to consider include other risk factors for cardiovascular disease, patient readiness for change, social support and community resources that support behavioral change, and other health care and preventive service priorities. Potential Harms: Harms may include the lost opportunity to provide other services with a greater health effect. Grade: C

Risk Assessment	If an individual's risk for cardiovascular disease is uncertain, there are several calculators and models available to quantify a person's 10-year risk for cardiac events, such as the Framingham-based Adult Treatment Panel III calculator (available at http://hp2010.nhlbihin.net/atpiii/calculator.asp). Generally, persons with a 10-year risk greater than 20% are considered to be high-risk, those with a 10-year risk less than 10% are considered to be low-risk, and those in the 10% to 20% range are considered to be intermediate-risk.
Interventions	Medium- or high-intensity behavioral interventions to promote a healthful diet and physical activity may be provided to individual patients in primary care settings or in other sectors of the health care system after referral from a primary care clinician. In addition, clinicians may offer healthful diet and physical activity interventions by referring the patient to community-based organizations. Strong linkages between the primary care setting and community-based resources may improve the delivery of these services.
Balance of Benefits and Harms	The USPSTF concludes with moderate certainty that medium- or high-intensity primary care behavioral counseling interventions to promote a healthful diet and physical activity have a small net benefit in adult patients without cardiovascular disease, hypertension, hyperlipidemia, or diabetes.
Other Relevant USPSTF Recommendations	The USPSTF has made recommendations on screening for carotid artery stenosis, coronary heart disease, high blood pressure, lipid disorders, peripheral arterial disease, and obesity. These recommendations are available at http://www.uspreventiveservicestaskforce.org/.

For a summary of the evidence systematically reviewed in making this recommendation, the full recommendation statement, and supporting documents, please go to http://www.uspreventiveservicestaskforce.org/.

35

Hearing Loss in Older Adults

Title	Screening for Hearing Loss in Older Adults
Population	Asymptomatic adults aged 50 years or older
Recommendation	**No recommendation.** **Grade: I (Insufficient Evidence)**

Risk Assessment	Increasing age is the most important risk factor for hearing loss. Other risk factors include a history of exposure to loud noises or ototoxic agents, including occupational exposures, previous recurrent inner ear infections, genetic factors, and certain systemic diseases, such as diabetes.
Screening Tests	Various screening tests are used in primary care settings to detect hearing loss in adults, including: • Whispered voice test • Finger rub test • Watch tick test • Single-item screening (for example, asking "Do you have difficulty with your hearing?") • Multiple-item patient questionnaire (for example, Hearing Handicap Inventory for the Elderly—Screening Version) • Handheld audiometer
Interventions	Hearing aids can improve self-reported hearing, communication, and social functioning for some adults with age-related hearing loss.
Balance of Benefits and Harms	There is inadequate evidence to determine the balance of benefits and harms of screening for hearing loss in adults aged 50 years or older.

For a summary of the evidence systematically reviewed in making these recommendations, the full recommendation statement, and supporting documents, please go to http://www.uspreventiveservicestaskforce.org/.

Hemochromatosis

Title	Screening for Hemochromatosis
Population	Asymptomatic general population
Recommendation	**Do not screen for hereditary hemochromatosis.** **Grade: D**

Risk Assessment	Clinically recognized hereditary hemochromatosis is primarily associated with mutations on the hemochromatosis (*HFE*) gene. Although this is a relatively common mutation in the U.S. population, only a small subset will develop symptoms of hemochromatosis. An even smaller proportion of these individuals will develop advanced stages of clinical disease.
Screening Tests	Genetic screening for *HFE* mutations can accurately identify individuals at risk for hereditary hemochromatosis. However, identifying an individual with the genotypic predisposition does not accurately predict the future risk for disease manifestation.
Interventions	Therapeutic phlebotomy is the main treatment for hereditary hemochromatosis. Phlebotomy is generally thought to have few side effects.
Balance of Benefits and Harms	• Screening could lead to identification of a large number of individuals who possess the high-risk genotype but may never manifest the clinical disease. This may result in unnecessary surveillance and diagnostic procedures, labeling, anxiety, and, potentially, unnecessary treatments. • There is poor evidence that early therapeutic phlebotomy improves morbidity and mortality in individuals with screening-detected versus clinically-detected hemochromatosis. • The USPSTF concluded that the potential harms of genetic screening for hereditary hemochromatosis outweigh the potential benefits.
Other Relevant USPSTF Recommendations	The USPSTF has also made recommendations on genetic testing for mutations in the breast cancer susceptibility gene to predict breast and ovarian cancer susceptibility. These recommendations are available at http://www.uspreventiveservicestaskforce.org/.

For a summary of the evidence systematically reviewed in making this recommendation, the full recommendation statement, and supporting documents, please go to http://www.uspreventiveservicestaskforce.org/.

Hepatitis B Virus Infection (Pregnant Women)

Title	Screening for Hepatitis B Virus Infection in Pregnancy
Population	All pregnant women
Recommendation	Screen for hepatitis B virus (HBV) at the first prenatal visit. Grade: A

Screening Tests	Serologic identification of hepatitis B surface antigen (HBsAg). Reported sensitivity and specificity are greater than 98%.
Timing of Screening	Order HBsAg testing at the first prenatal visit. Re-screen women with unknown HBsAg status or new or continuing risk factors at admission to hospital, birth center, or other delivery setting.
Interventions	Administer hepatitis B vaccine and hepatitis B immune globulin to HBV-exposed infants within 12 hours of birth. Refer women who test positive for counseling and medical management. Counseling should include information about how to prevent transmission to sexual partners and household contacts. Reassure patients that breastfeeding is safe for infants who receive appropriate prophylaxis.
Implementation	Establish systems for timely transfer of maternal HBsAg test results to the labor and delivery and newborn medical records.
Other Relevant USPSTF Recommendations	USPSTF recommendations on the screening of pregnant women for other infections, including asymptomatic bacteriuria, bacterial vaginosis, chlamydia, HIV, and syphilis, can be found at http://www.uspreventiveservicestaskforce.org.

For a summary of the evidence systematically reviewed in making these recommendations, the full recommendation statement, and supporting documents, please go to http://www.uspreventiveservicestaskforce.org.

Hepatitis C Virus Infection

Title	Screening for Hepatitis C Virus Infection in Adults
Population	Persons at high risk for infection and adults born between 1945 and 1965
Recommendation	Screen for hepatitis C virus (HCV) infection. Grade: B

Risk Assessment	The most important risk factor for HCV infection is past or current injection drug use. Additional risk factors include receiving a blood transfusion before 1992, long-term hemodialysis, being born to an HCV-infected mother, incarceration, intranasal drug use, getting an unregulated tattoo, and other percutaneous exposures. Adults born between 1945 and 1965 are more likely to be diagnosed with HCV infection, either because they received a blood transfusion before the introduction of screening in 1992 or because they have a history of other risk factors for exposure decades earlier.
Screening Tests	Anti-HCV antibody testing followed by confirmatory polymerase chain reaction testing accurately identifies patients with chronic HCV infection. Various noninvasive tests with good diagnostic accuracy are possible alternatives to liver biopsy for diagnosing fibrosis or cirrhosis.
Screening Interval	Persons with continued risk for HCV infection (such as injection drug users) should be screened periodically. Evidence on how often screening should occur in these persons is lacking. Adults born between 1945 and 1965 and persons who are at risk because of potential exposure before universal blood screening need only be screened once.
Treatment	Antiviral treatment prevents long-term health complications of HCV infection (such as cirrhosis, liver failure, and hepatocellular carcinoma). The combination of pegylated interferon (α-2a or α-2b) and ribavirin is the standard treatment for HCV infection. In 2011, the U.S. Food and Drug Administration approved the protease inhibitors boceprevir and telaprevir for the treatment of HCV genotype 1 infection (the predominant genotype in the United States).
Balance of Benefits and Harms	On the basis of the accuracy of HCV antibody testing and the availability of effective interventions for persons with HCV infection, the USPSTF concludes that there is a moderate net benefit to screening in populations at high risk for infection. The USPSTF concludes that there is also a moderate net benefit to 1-time screening in all adults in the United States born between 1945 and 1965.
Other Relevant USPSTF Recommendations	The USPSTF has made recommendations on screening for hepatitis B virus infection in adolescents, adults, and pregnant women. These recommendations are available at http://www.uspreventiveservicestaskforce.org/.

For a summary of the evidence systematically reviewed in making this recommendation, the full recommendation statement, and supporting documents, please go to http://www.uspreventiveservicestaskforce.org/.

High Blood Pressure in Adults

Title	Screening for High Blood Pressure in adults
Population	Adult general population[1]
Recommendation	Screen for high blood pressure. Grade: A

Screening Tests	High blood pressure (hypertension) is usually defined in adults as: systolic blood pressure (SBP) of 140 mm Hg or higher, or diastolic blood pressure (DBP) of 90 mm Hg or higher. Due to variability in individual blood pressure measurements, it is recommended that hypertension be diagnosed only after 2 or more elevated readings are obtained on at least 2 visits over a period of 1 to several weeks.
Screening Intervals	The optimal interval for screening adults for hypertension is not known. The Joint National Committee on Prevention, Detection, Evaluation, and Treatment of High Blood Pressure (JNC 7) recommends: • Screening every 2 years with BP <120/80. • Screening every year with SBP of 120-139 mmHg or DBP of 80-90 mmHg.
Treatment	A variety of pharmacological agents are available to treat hypertension. JNC 7 guidelines for treatment of hypertension can be accessed at http://www.nhlbi.nih.gov/guidelines/hypertension/jncintro.htm. The following non-pharmacological therapies are associated with reductions in blood pressure: • Reduction of dietary sodium intake. • Potassium supplementation. • Increased physical activity, weight loss. • Stress management. • Reduction of alcohol intake.
Other Relevant USPSTF Recommendations	Adults with hypertension should be screened for diabetes. Adults should be screened for hyperlipidemia (depending on age, sex, risk factors) and smoking. Clinicians should discuss aspirin chemoprevention with patients at increased risk for cardiovascular disease. These recommendations and related evidence are available at http://www.uspreventiveservicestaskforce.org.

[1]This recommendation applies to adults without known hypertension.

For a summary of the evidence systematically reviewed in making these recommendations, the full recommendation statement, and supporting documents, please go to http://www.uspreventiveservicestaskforce.org.

HIV Infection

Title	Screening for HIV
Population	Adolescents and adults aged 15 to 65 years, younger adolescents and older adults at increased risk for infection, and pregnant women
Recommendation	Screen for HIV infection. Grade: A

Risk Assessment	Men who have sex with men and active injection drug users are at very high risk for new HIV infection. Other persons at high risk include those who have acquired or request testing for other sexually transmitted infections. Behavioral risk factors for HIV infection include: • Having unprotected vaginal or anal intercourse • Having sexual partners who are HIV-infected, bisexual, or injection drug users • Exchanging sex for drugs or money The USPSTF recognizes that the above categories are not mutually exclusive, the degree of sexual risk is on a continuum, and individuals may not be aware of their sexual partners' risk factors for HIV infection.
Screening Tests	The conventional serum test for diagnosing HIV infection is repeatedly reactive immunoassay, followed by confirmatory Western blot or immunofluorescent assay. Conventional HIV test results are available within 1 to 2 days from most commercial laboratories. Rapid HIV testing may use either blood or oral fluid specimens and can provide results in 5 to 40 minutes; however, initial positive results require confirmation with conventional methods. Other U.S. Food and Drug Administration–approved tests for detection and confirmation of HIV infection include combination tests (for p24 antigen and HIV antibodies) and qualitative HIV-1 RNA.
Interventions	At present, there is no cure for chronic HIV infection. However, appropriately timed interventions in HIV-positive persons can reduce risks for clinical progression, complications or death from the disease, and disease transmission. Effective interventions include antiretroviral therapy (ART) (specifically, the use of combined ART), immunizations, and prophylaxis for opportunistic infections.
Balance of Benefits and Harms	The net benefit of screening for HIV infection in adolescents, adults, and pregnant women is substantial.
Other Relevant USPSTF Recommendations	The USPSTF has made recommendations on behavioral counseling to prevent sexually transmitted infections. This recommendation is available at http://www.uspreventiveservicestaskforce.org/.

For a summary of the evidence systematically reviewed in making this recommendation, the full recommendation statement, and supporting documents, please go to http://www.uspreventiveservicestaskforce.org/.

Illicit Drug Use

Title	Screening for Illicit Drug Use
Population	Adolescents[1], adults, and pregnant women not previously identified as users of illicit drugs
Recommendation	No recommendation. Grade I: (Insufficient Evidence)

Screening Tests	Toxicologic tests of blood or urine can provide objective evidence of drug use, but do not distinguish occasional users from impaired drug users. Valid and reliable standardized questionnaires are available to screen adolescents and adults for drug use or misuse. There is insufficient evidence to evaluate the clinical utility of these instruments when widely applied in primary care settings.
Balance of Benefits and Harms	The USPSTF concludes that for adolescents, adults, and pregnant women, the evidence is insufficient to determine the benefits and harms of screening for illicit drug use.
Suggestions for Practice	Clinicians should be alert to the signs and symptoms of illicit drug use in patients.
Treatment	More evidence is needed on the effectiveness of primary care office-based treatments for illicit drug use/dependence.
Other Relevant USPSTF Recommendations	The USPSTF recommendation for screening and counseling interventions to reduce alcohol misuse by adults and pregnant women can be found at http://www.uspreventiveservicestaskforce.org/uspstf/uspsdrin.htm.

[1]For adolescents, see also Illicit and Prescription Drug Use in Children and Adolescents, Counseling

For a summary of the evidence systematically reviewed in making these recommendations, the full recommendation statement, and supporting documents, please go to http://www.uspreventiveservicestaskforce.org.

Impaired Visual Acuity in Older Adults[1]

Title	Screening for Impaired Visual Acuity in Older Adults[1]
Population	Adults age 65 and older
Recommendation	No recommendation. Grade: I (Insufficient Evidence)

Risk Assessment	Older age is an important risk factor for most types of visual impairment. Additional risk factors include: • Smoking, alcohol use, exposure to ultraviolet light, diabetes, corticosteroids, and black race (for cataracts). • Smoking, family history, and white race (for age-related macular degeneration).
Screening Tests	Visual acuity testing (for example, the Snellen eye chart) is the usual method for screening for impairment of visual acuity in the primary care setting. Screening questions are not as accurate as a visual acuity test.
Balance of Benefits and Harms	There is no direct evidence that screening for vision impairment in older adults in primary care settings is associated with improved clinical outcomes. There is evidence that early treatment of refractive error, cataracts, and age-related macular degeneration may lead to harms that are small. The magnitude of net benefit for screening cannot be calculated because of a lack of evidence.
Other Relevant USPSTF Recommendations	Recommendations on screening for glaucoma and on screening for hearing loss in older adults can be accessed at http://www.uspreventiveservicestaskforce.org.

[1]This recommendation does not cover screening for glaucoma.

For a summary of the evidence systematically reviewed in making these recommendations, the full recommendation statement, and supporting documents, please go to http://www.uspreventiveservicestaskforce.org.

Intimate Partner Violence and Elderly Abuse

Title	Screening for Intimate Partner Violence and Abuse of Elderly and Vulnerable Adults	
Population	Asymptomatic women of childbearing age	Elderly or vulnerable adults
Recommendation	Screen women for intimate partner violence (IPV), and provide or refer women who screen positive to intervention services. Grade: B	No recommendation. Grade: I (Insufficient Evidence)

Risk Assessment	While all women are at potential risk for abuse, factors that elevate risk include young age, substance abuse, marital difficulties, and economic hardships.	
Interventions	Adequate evidence from randomized trials support a variety of interventions for women of childbearing age that can be delivered or referred by primary care, including counseling, home visits, information cards, referrals to community services, and mentoring support. Depending on the type of intervention, these services may be provided by clinicians, nurses, social workers, nonclinician mentors, or community workers.	
Balance of Benefits and Harms	Screening and interventions for IPV in women of childbearing age are associated with moderate health improvements through the reduction of exposure to abuse, physical and mental harms, and mortality. The associated harms are deemed no greater than small. Therefore, the overall net benefit is moderate.	The USPSTF was not able to estimate the magnitude of net benefit for screening all elderly or vulnerable adults (i.e., adults who are physically or mentally dysfunctional) for abuse and neglect because there were no studies on the accuracy, effectiveness, or harms of screening in this population.
Other Relevant USPSTF Recommendations	The USPSTF has made recommendations on screening for depression in adults and screening and counseling to reduce alcohol misuse in adults. These recommendations are available at http://www.uspreventiveservicestaskforce.org/.	

For a summary of the evidence systematically reviewed in making this recommendation, the full recommendation statement, and supporting documents, please go to http://www.uspreventiveservicestaskforce.org/.

Lipid Disorders in Adults

Title	Screening for Lipid Disorders in Adults	
Population	• Men age 35 years and older • Women age 45 years and older who are at increased risk for coronary heart disease (CHD)	• Men ages 20 to 35 years who are at increased risk for CHD • Women ages 20 to 45 years who are at increased risk for CHD	• Men ages 20 to 35 years • Women ages 20 years and older who are not at increased risk for CHD
Recommendation	Screen for lipid disorders. **Grade: A**	Screen for lipid disorders. **Grade: B**	No recommendation for or against screening **Grade: C**
Risk Assessment	Consideration of lipid levels along with other risk factors allows for an accurate estimation of CHD risk. Risk factors for CHD include diabetes, history of previous CHD or atherosclerosis, family history of cardiovascular disease, tobacco use, hypertension, and obesity (body mass index ≥30 kg/m²).		
Screening Tests	The preferred screening tests for dyslipidemia are measuring serum lipid (total cholesterol, high-density and low-denisty lipoprotein cholesterol) levels in non-fasting or fasting samples. Abnormal screening results should be confirmed by a repeated sample on a separate occasion, and the average of both results should be used for risk assessment.		
Timing of Screening	The optimal interval for screening is uncertain. Reasonable options include every 5 years, shorter intervals for people who have lipid levels close to those warranting therapy, and longer intervals for those not at increased risk who have had repeatedly normal lipid levels. An age at which to stop screening has not been established. Screening may be appropriate in older people who have never been screened; repeated screening is less important in older people because lipid levels are less likely to increase after age 65 years.		
Interventions	Drug therapy is usually more effective than diet alone in improving lipid profiles, but choice of treatment should consider overall risk, costs of treatment, and patient preferences. Guidelines for treating lipid disorders are available from the National Cholesterol Education Program of the National Institutes of Health (http://www.nhlbi.nih.gov/about/ncep/).		
Balance of Benefits and Harms	The benefits of screening for and treating lipid disorders in men age 35 and older and women age 45 and older at increased risk for CHD substantially outweigh the potential harms.	The benefits of screening for and treating lipid disorders in young adults at increased risk for CHD moderately outweigh the potential harms.	The net benefits of screening for lipid disorders in young adults not at increased risk for CHD are not sufficient to make a general recommendation.
Other Relevant USPSTF Recommendations	The USPSTF has made recommendations on screening for lipid disorders in children and screening for carotid artery stenosis, coronary heart disease, high blood pressure, and peripheral arterial disease. These recommendations are available at http://www.uspreventiveservicestaskforce.org/.		

For a summary of the evidence systematically reviewed in making this recommendation, the full recommendation statement, and supporting documents, please go to http://www.uspreventiveservicestaskforce.org/.

Lung Cancer

Title	Screening for Lung Cancer
Population	Asymptomatic adults aged 55 to 80 years who have a 30 pack-year smoking history and currently smoke or have quit smoking within the past 15 years
Recommendation	**Screen annually for lung cancer with low-dose computed tomography.** **Discontinue screening when the patient has not smoked for 15 years.** **Grade: B**

Risk Assessment	Age, total cumulative exposure to tobacco smoke, and years since quitting smoking are the most important risk factors for lung cancer. Other risk factors include specific occupational exposures, radon exposure, family history, and history of pulmonary fibrosis or chronic obstructive lung disease.
Screening Tests	Low-dose computed tomography has high sensitivity and acceptable specificity for detecting lung cancer in high-risk persons and is the only currently recommended screening test for lung cancer.
Treatment	Non–small cell lung cancer is treated with surgical resection when possible and also with radiation and chemotherapy.
Balance of Benefits and Harms	Annual screening for lung cancer with low-dose computed tomography is of moderate net benefit in asymptomatic persons who are at high risk for lung cancer based on age, total cumulative exposure to tobacco smoke, and years since quitting smoking.
Other Relevant USPSTF Recommendations	The USPSTF has made recommendations on counseling and interventions to prevent tobacco use and tobacco-caused disease. These recommendations are available at http://www.uspreventiveservicestaskforce.org/.

For a summary of the evidence systematically reviewed in making this recommendation, the full recommendation statement, and supporting documents, please go to http://www.uspreventiveservicestaskforce.org/.

Menopausal Hormone Therapy

Title	Menopausal Hormone Therapy for the Primary Prevention of Chronic Conditions	
Population	Postmenopausal women	Postmenopausal women who have had a hysterectomy
Recommendation	Do not prescribe combined estrogen and progestin for the prevention of chronic conditions. Grade: D	Do not prescribe estrogen for the prevention of chronic conditions. Grade: D

Risk Assessment	This recommendation applies to the average-risk population. Risk factors for a specific chronic disease or individual characteristics that affect the likelihood of a specific therapy-associated adverse event may cause a woman's net balance of benefits and harms to differ from that of the average population.
Preventive Medications	Although combined estrogen and progestin therapy (specifically, oral conjugated equine estrogen, 0.625 mg/d, plus medroxyprogesterone acetate, 2.5 mg/d) decreases the risk for fractures in postmenopausal women, there is an accompanying increased risk for serious adverse events, such as stroke, invasive breast cancer, dementia, gallbladder disease, deep venous thrombosis, and pulmonary embolism. Estrogen therapy (specifically, oral conjugated equine estrogen, 0.625 mg/d) decreases the risk for fractures and has a small effect on the risk for invasive breast cancer, but it is also associated with important harms, such as an increased likelihood of stroke, deep venous thrombosis, and gallbladder disease. Neither combined estrogen and progestin therapy nor estrogen alone reduces the risk for coronary heart disease in postmenopausal women.
Balance of Benefits and Harms	The chronic disease prevention benefits of combined estrogen and progestin do not outweigh the harms in most postmenopausal women.	The chronic disease prevention benefits of estrogen are unlikely to outweigh the harms in most postmenopausal women who have had a hysterectomy.
Other Relevant USPSTF Recommendations	The USPSTF has made recommendations on screening for osteoporosis and the use of preventive medications for breast cancer, as well as other relevant interventions for the primary or secondary prevention of chronic diseases in women, such as medications for cardiovascular disease and screening for coronary heart disease, high blood pressure, lipid disorders, colorectal cancer, breast cancer, and dementia. These recommendations are available at http://www.uspreventiveservicestaskforce.org/.	

For a summary of the evidence systematically reviewed in making this recommendation, the full recommendation statement, and supporting documents, please go to http://www.uspreventiveservicestaskforce.org/.

Motor Vehicle Occupant Restraints

Title	Primary Care Counseling for Proper Use of Motor Vehicle Occupant Restraints
Population	General primary care population
Recommendation	**No recommendation.** **Grade: I (Insufficient Evidence)**

Interventions	There is good evidence that community and public health interventions, including legislation, law enforcement campaigns, car seat distribution campaigns, media campaigns, and other community-based interventions, are effective in improving the proper use of car seats, booster seats, and seat belts.
Suggestions for Practice	Current evidence is insufficient to assess the incremental benefit of counseling in primary care settings, beyond increases related to other interventions, in improving rates of proper use of motor vehicle occupant restraints. Linkages between primary care and community interventions are critical for improving proper car seat, booster seat, and seat belt use.
Relevant Recommendations from the Guide to Community Preventive Services	The Community Preventive Services Task Force has reviewed evidence of the effectiveness of selected population-based interventions to reduce motor vehicle occupant injuries, focusing on three strategic areas: • Increasing the proper use of child safety seats. • Increasing the use of safety belts. • Reducing alcohol-impaired driving. Multiple interventions in these areas have been recommended. Recommendations can be accessed at http://www.thecommunityguide.org/mvoi/

For a summary of the evidence systematically reviewed in making these recommendations, the full recommendation statement, and supporting documents, please go to http://www.uspreventiveservicestaskforce.org.

Obesity in Adults

Title	Screening for and Management Of Obesity In Adults
Population	Adults aged 18 years or older
Recommendation	Screen for obesity. Patients with a body mass index (BMI) of 30 kg/m² or higher should be offered or referred to intensive, multicomponent behavioral interventions. Grade: B

Screening Tests	Body mass index is calculated from the measured weight and height of an individual. Recent evidence suggests that waist circumference may be an acceptable alternative to BMI measurement in some patient subpopulations.
Timing of Screening	No evidence was found about appropriate intervals for screening.
Interventions	Intensive, multicomponent behavioral interventions for obese adults include the following components: • Behavioral management activities, such as setting weight-loss goals • Improving diet or nutrition and increasing physical activity • Addressing barriers to change • Self-monitoring • Strategizing how to maintain lifestyle changes
Balance of Benefits and Harms	Adequate evidence indicates that intensive, multicomponent behavioral interventions for obese adults can lead to weight loss, as well as improved glucose tolerance and other physiologic risk factors for cardiovascular disease. Inadequate evidence was found about the effectiveness of these interventions on long-term health outcomes (for example, mortality, cardiovascular disease, and hospitalizations). Adequate evidence indicates that the harms of screening and behavioral interventions for obesity are small. Possible harms of behavioral weight-loss interventions include decreased bone mineral density and increased fracture risk, serious injuries resulting from increased physical activity, and increased risk for eating disorders.
Other relevant USPSTF recommendations	Recommendations on screening for obesity in children and adolescents can be found at http://www.uspreventiveservicestaskforce.org/.

For a summary of the evidence systematically reviewed in making this recommendation, the full recommendation statement, and supporting documents, please go to http://www.uspreventiveserviceservicestaskforce.org/.

49

Oral Cancer

Title	Screening for Oral Cancer
Population	Asymptomatic adults aged 18 years or older
Recommendation	No recommendation. Grade: I (Insufficient Evidence)

Risk Assessment	The primary risk factors for oral cancer are tobacco and alcohol use. Additional risk factors include male sex, older age, use of betel quid, ultraviolet light exposure, infection with *Candida* or bacterial flora, and a compromised immune system. Recently, sexually transmitted oral human papillomavirus infection has been recognized as an increasing risk factor for oropharyngeal cancer, another subset of head and neck cancer.
Screening Tests	The primary screening test for oral cancer is a systematic clinical examination, including inspection and palpation of the oral cavity.
Treatment	Suspected oral cancer or its precursors detected on examination require confirmation by tissue biopsy. Treatment for screen-detected oral cancer includes surgery, radiotherapy, and chemotherapy.
Balance of Benefits and Harms	The USPSTF found inadequate evidence on the diagnostic accuracy, benefits, and harms of screening for oral cancer. Therefore, the USPSTF cannot determine the balance of benefits and harms of screening for oral cancer in asymptomatic adults.
Other Relevant USPSTF Recommendations	The USPSTF has made recommendations on counseling to prevent tobacco use and screening for and counseling to reduce alcohol misuse. These recommendations are available at http://www.uspreventiveservicestaskforce.org/.

For a summary of the evidence systematically reviewed in making this recommendation, the full recommendation statement, and supporting documents, please go to http://www.uspreventiveservicestaskforce.org/.

50

Osteoporosis

Title	Screening for Osteoporosis	
Population	Women age ≥65 years without previous known fractures or secondary causes of osteoporosis	Women age <65 years whose 10-year fracture risk is equal to or greater than that of a 65-year-old white woman without additional risk factors	Men without previous known fractures or secondary causes of osteoporosis
Recommendation	Screen for osteoporosis. Grade: B		No recommendation. Grade: I (Insufficient Evidence)

Risk Assessment	As many as 1 in 2 postmenopausal women and 1 in 5 older men are at risk for an osteoporosis-related fracture. Osteoporosis is common in all racial groups but is most common in white persons. Rates of osteoporosis increase with age. Elderly people are particularly susceptible to fractures. According to the FRAX fracture risk assessment tool, available at http://www.shef.ac.uk/FRAX/, the 10-year fracture risk in a 65-year-old white woman without additional risk factors is 9.3%.
Screening Tests	Current diagnostic and treatment criteria rely on dual-energy x-ray absorptiometry of the hip and lumbar spine.
Timing of Screening	Evidence is lacking about optimal intervals for repeated screening.
Intervention	In addition to adequate calcium and vitamin D intake and weight-bearing exercise, multiple U.S. Food and Drug Administration–approved therapies reduce fracture risk in women with low bone mineral density and no previous fractures, including bisphosphonates, parathyroid hormone, raloxifene, and estrogen. The choice of treatment should take into account the patient's clinical situation and the tradeoff between benefits and harms. Clinicians should provide education about how to minimize drug side effects.
Suggestions for Practice Regarding the I Statement for Men	Clinicians should consider: • potential preventable burden: increasing because of the aging of the U.S. population • potential harms: likely to be small, mostly opportunity costs • current practice: routine screening of men not widespread • costs: additional scanners required to screen sizeable populations Men most likely to benefit from screening have a 10-year risk for osteoporotic fracture equal to or greater than that of a 65-year-old white woman without risk factors. However, current evidence is insufficient to assess the balance of benefits and harms of screening for osteoporosis in men.

For a summary of the evidence systematically reviewed in making these recommendations, the full recommendation statement, and supporting documents, please go to http://www.uspreventiveservicestaskforce.org.

51

Ovarian Cancer

Title	Screening for Ovarian Cancer
Population	Asymptomatic women without known genetic mutations that increase risk for ovarian cancer
Recommendation	Do not screen for ovarian cancer. Grade: D

Risk Assessment	Women with *BRCA1* and *BRCA2* genetic mutations, the Lynch syndrome (hereditary nonpolyposis colon cancer), or a family history of ovarian cancer are at increased risk for ovarian cancer. Women with an increased-risk family history should be considered for genetic counseling to further evaluate their potential risks. "Increased-risk family history" generally means having 2 or more first- or second-degree relatives with a history of ovarian cancer or a combination of breast and ovarian cancer; for women of Ashkenazi Jewish descent, it means having a first-degree relative (or 2 second-degree relatives on the same side of the family) with breast or ovarian cancer.
Screening Tests	Transvaginal ultrasonography and serum cancer antigen (CA)–125 testing are the most commonly suggested screening modalities.
Treatments	Treatment of ovarian carcinoma includes surgical treatment (debulking) and intraperitoneal or systemic chemotherapy.
Balance of Benefits and Harms	Annual screening with transvaginal ultrasonography and serum CA-125 testing in women does not decrease ovarian cancer mortality. Screening for ovarian cancer can lead to important harms, including major surgical interventions in women who do not have cancer. Therefore, the harms of screening for ovarian cancer outweigh the benefits.
Other Relevant USPSTF Recommendations	The USPSTF has made a recommendation on genetic risk assessment and BRCA mutation testing for breast and ovarian cancer susceptibility. This recommendation is available at http://www.uspreventiveservicestaskforce.org/.

For a summary of the evidence systematically reviewed in making this recommendation, the full recommendation statement, and supporting documents, please go to http://www.uspreventiveservicestaskforce.org/.

Peripheral Artery Disease

Title	**Screening for Peripheral Artery Disease and Cardiovascular Disease Risk Assessment with the Ankle Brachial Index in Adults**
Population	Asymptomatic adults without a known diagnosis of peripheral artery disease (PAD), cardiovascular disease, severe chronic kidney disease, or diabetes
Recommendation	**No recommendation.** **Grade: I (Insufficient Evidence)**

Risk Assessment	Important risk factors for PAD include older age, diabetes, smoking, hypertension, high cholesterol level, obesity, and physical inactivity. Peripheral artery disease is more common in men than women and occurs at an earlier age in men.
Screening Tests	Resting ankle–brachial index (ABI) is the most commonly used test in screening for and detection of PAD in clinical settings. It is calculated as the systolic blood pressure obtained at the ankle divided by the systolic blood pressure obtained at the brachial artery while the patient is lying down. Physical examination has low sensitivity for detecting mild PAD in asymptomatic persons.
Balance of Benefits and Harms	Evidence on screening for PAD with the ABI in asymptomatic adults with no known diagnosis of cardiovascular disease or diabetes is insufficient; therefore, the balance of benefits and harms cannot be determined.
Other Relevant USPSTF Recommendations	The USPSTF has made recommendations on using nontraditional risk factors, including the ABI, in screening for coronary heart disease. These recommendations are available at http://www.uspreventiveservicestaskforce.org/.

For a summary of the evidence systematically reviewed in making this recommendation, the full recommendation statement, and supporting documents, please go to http://www.uspreventiveservicestaskforce.org/.

Prostate Cancer

Title	**Screening for Prostate Cancer**
Population	Adult males
Recommendation	**Do not use prostate-specific antigen (PSA)-based screening for prostate cancer.** **Grade: D**

Screening Tests	Contemporary recommendations for prostate cancer screening all incorporate the measurement of serum PSA levels; other methods of detection, such as digital rectal examination or ultrasonography, may be included. There is convincing evidence that PSA-based screening programs result in the detection of many cases of asymptomatic prostate cancer, and that a substantial percentage of men who have asymptomatic cancer detected by PSA screening have a tumor that either will not progress or will progress so slowly that it would have remained asymptomatic for the man's lifetime (i.e., PSA-based screening results in considerable overdiagnosis).
Interventions	Management strategies for localized prostate cancer include watchful waiting, active surveillance, surgery, and radiation therapy. There is no consensus regarding optimal treatment.
Balance of Benefits and Harms	The reduction in prostate cancer mortality 10 to 14 years after PSA-based screening is, at most, very small, even for men in the optimal age range of 55 to 69 years. The harms of screening include pain, fever, bleeding, infection, and transient urinary difficulties associated with prostate biopsy, psychological harm of false-positive test results, and overdiagnosis. Harms of treatment include erectile dysfunction, urinary incontinence, bowel dysfunction, and a small risk for premature death. Because of the current inability to reliably distinguish tumors that will remain indolent from those destined to be lethal, many men are being subjected to the harms of treatment for prostate cancer that will never become symptomatic. The benefits of PSA-based screening for prostate cancer do not outweigh the harms.
Relevant USPSTF Recommendations	Recommendations on screening for other types of cancer can be found at http://www.uspreventiveservicestaskforce.org/.

For a summary of the evidence systematically reviewed in making these recommendations, the full recommendation statement, and supporting documents, please go to http://www.uspreventiveservicestaskforce.org/.

Sexually Transmitted Infections

Title	Behavioral Counseling to Prevent Sexually Transmitted Infections		
Population	All sexually active adolescents	Adults at increased risk for STIs	Non-sexually-active adolescents and adults not at increased risk for STIs
Recommendation	Offer high-intensity counseling. Grade: B	Offer high-intensity counseling. Grade: B	No recommendation. Grade: I (Insufficient Evidence)
Risk Assessment	All sexually active adolescents are at increased risk for STIs and should be offered counseling. Adults should be considered at increased risk and offered counseling if they have: • Current STIs or have had an STI within the past year. • Multiple sexual partners. In communities or populations with high rates of STIs, all sexually active patients in non-monogamous relationships may be considered at increased risk.		
Interventions	Characteristics of successful high-intensity counseling interventions: • Multiple sessions of counseling. • Frequently delivered in group settings.		
Suggestions for Practice	High-intensity counseling may be delivered in primary care settings, or in other sectors of the health system and community settings after referral. Delivery of this service may be greatly improved by strong linkages between the primary care setting and community.		Evidence is limited regarding counseling for adolescents who are not sexually active. Intensive counseling for all adolescents in order to reach those who are at risk but have not been appropriately identified is not supported by current evidence. Evidence is lacking regarding the effectiveness of counseling for adults not at increased risk for STIs.
Other Relevant USPSTF Recommendations	USPSTF recommendations on screening for chlamydial infection, gonorrhea, genital herpes, hepatitis B, hepatitis C, HIV, and syphilis can be found at http://www.uspreventiveservicestaskforce.org.		

Abbreviation: STI = Sexually Transmitted Infection

For a summary of the evidence systematically reviewed in making these recommendations, the full recommendation statement, and supporting documents, please go to http://www.uspreventiveservicestaskforce.org.

Skin Cancer (Counseling)

Title	Behavioral Counseling to Prevent Skin Cancer	
Population	Children, adolescents, and young adults aged 10 to 24 years with fair skin	Adults older than age 24 years
Recommendation	Provide counseling about minimizing exposure to ultraviolet radiation to reduce risk for skin cancer. Grade: B	No recommendation. Grade: I (Insufficient Evidence)

Risk Assessment	Individuals with a fair skin type are at greatly increased risk for skin cancer. Fair skin type can be defined by eye and hair color; freckling; and historical factors, such as usual reaction to sun exposure (always or usually burning or infrequently tanning).
Behavioral Counseling	Effective counseling interventions were generally of low intensity and almost entirely accomplished within the primary care visit. Successful counseling interventions used cancer prevention or appearance-focused messages (such as stressing the aging effect of ultraviolet radiation on the skin) to reach specific audiences.
Interventions	Behavior change interventions are aimed at reducing ultraviolet radiation exposure. Sun-protective behaviors include the use of a broad-spectrum sunscreen with a sun protection factor ≥ 15, wearing hats or other shade-protective clothing, avoiding the outdoors during midday hours (10 a.m. to 3 p.m.), and avoiding the use of indoor tanning.
Balance of Benefits and Harms	For children, adolescents, and young adults aged 10 to 24 years with fair skin, primary care counseling interventions can increase the use of sun-protective behaviors by a moderate amount, with no appreciable harms. For adults older than 24 years, there is inadequate evidence to determine the effect of counseling on the use of sun-protective behaviors.
Other Relevant USPSTF Recommendations	The USPSTF has made recommendations on screening for skin cancer. These recommendations are available at http://www.uspreventiveservicestaskforce.org/.

For a summary of the evidence systematically reviewed in making this recommendation, the full recommendation statement, and supporting documents, please go to http://www.uspreventiveservicestaskforce.org/.

Skin Cancer (Screening)

Title	Screening for Skin Cancer
Population	Adult general population[1]
Recommendation	No recommendation. Grade: I (Insufficient Evidence)

Risk Assessment	Skin cancer risks: family history of skin cancer, considerable history of sun exposure and sunburn. Groups at increased risk for melanoma: • Fair-skinned men and women over the age of 65 years. • Patients with atypical moles. • Patients with more than 50 moles.
Screening Tests	There is insufficient evidence to assess the balance of benefits and harms of whole body skin examination by a clinician or patient skin self-examination for the early detection of skin cancer.
Screening Intervals	Not applicable.
Suggestions for Practice	Clinicians should remain alert for skin lesions with malignant features that are noted while performing physical examinations for other purposes. Features associated with increased risk for malignancy include: asymmetry, border irregularity, color variability, diameter >6mm ("A," "B," "C," "D"), or rapidly changing lesions. Suspicious lesions should be biopsied.
Other Relevant Recommendations from the USPSTF and the Community Preventive Services Task Force	The USPSTF has reviewed the evidence for counseling to prevent skin cancer. The recommendation statement and supporting documents can be accessed at http://www.uspreventiveservicestaskforce.org. The Community Preventive Services Task Force has reviewed the evidence on public health interventions to reduce skin cancer. The recommendations can be accessed at http://www.thecommunityguide.org.

[1]The USPSTF does not examine outcomes related to surveillance of patients with familial syndromes, such as familial atypical mole and melanoma (FAM-M) syndrome.

For a summary of the evidence systematically reviewed in making these recommendations, the full recommendation statement, and supporting documents, please go to http://www.uspreventiveservicestaskforce.org.

Suicide Risk

Title	Screening for Suicide Risk
Population	General population
Recommendation	No recommendation. Grade: I (Insufficient Evidence)

Risk Assessment	The strongest risk factors for attempted suicide include mood disorders or other mental disorders, comorbid substance abuse disorders, history of deliberate self-harm, and a history of suicide attempts. Deliberate self-harm refers to intentionally initiated acts of self-harm with a nonfatal outcome (including self-poisoning and self-injury). Suicide risk is assessed along a continuum ranging from suicidal ideation alone (relatively less severe) to suicidal ideation with a plan (more severe). Suicidal ideation with a specific plan of action is associated with a significant risk for attempted suicide.
Screening Tests	There is limited evidence on the accuracy of screening tools to identify suicide risk in the primary care setting, including tools to identify those at high risk. The characteristics of the most commonly used screening instruments (Scale for Suicide Ideation, Scale for Suicide Ideation—Worst, and the Suicidal Ideation Questionnaire) have not been validated to assess suicide risk in primary care settings.
Interventions	There is insufficient evidence to determine if treatment of persons at high risk for suicide reduces suicide attempts or mortality.
Balance of Benefits and Harms	There is no evidence that screening for suicide risk reduces suicide attempts or mortality. There is insufficient evidence to determine if treatment of persons at high risk reduces suicide attempts or mortality. There are no studies that directly address the harms of screening and treatment for suicide risk. As a result, the USPSTF could not determine the balance of benefits and harms of screening for suicide risk in the primary care setting.
Other Relevant USPSTF Recommendations	The USPSTF has also made recommendations on screening for alcohol misuse, depression, and illicit drug use. These recommendations are available at http://www.uspreventiveservicestaskforce.org/.

For a summary of the evidence systematically reviewed in making this recommendation, the full recommendation statement, and supporting documents, please go to http://www.uspreventiveservicestaskforce.org/.

Syphilis (Pregnant Women)

Title	Screening for Syphilis Infection in Pregnancy
Population	All pregnant women
Recommendation	Screen for syphilis infection. Grade: A

Screening Tests	Nontreponemal tests commonly used for initial screening include: • Venereal Disease Research Laboratory (VDRL) • Rapid Plasma Reagin (RPR) Confirmatory tests include: • Fluorescent treponemal antibody absorbed (FTA-ABS) • *Treponema pallidum* particle agglutination (TPPA)
Timing of Screening	Test all pregnant women at the first prenatal visit.
Other Clinical Considerations	Most organizations recommend testing high-risk women again during the third trimester and at delivery. Groups at increased risk include: • Uninsured women • Women living in poverty • Sex workers • Illicit drug users • Those diagnosed with other sexually transmitted infections (STIs) • Other women living in communities with high syphilis morbidity Prevalence is higher in southern U.S. and in metropolitan areas and in Hispanic and African American populations.
Interventions	The Centers for Disease Control and Prevention (CDC) recommends treatment with parenteral benzathine penicillin G. Women with penicillin allergies should be desensitized and treated with penicillin. Consult the CDC for the most up-to-date recommendations: http://www.cdc.gov/std/treatment/.
Other Relevant USPSTF Recommendations	Recommendations on screening for other STIs, and on counseling for STIs, can be found at http://www.uspreventiveservicestaskforce.org.

For a summary of the evidence systematically reviewed in making these recommendations, the full recommendation statement, and supporting documents, please go to http://www.uspreventiveservicestaskforce.org.

Testicular Cancer

Title	Screening for Testicular Cancer
Population	Adolescent and adult males
Recommendation	Do not screen. Grade: D

Screening Tests	There is inadequate evidence that screening asymptomatic patients by means of self-examination or clinician examination has greater yield or accuracy for detecting testicular cancer at more curable stages.
Interventions	Management of testicular cancer consists of orchiectomy and may include other surgery, radiation therapy, or chemotherapy, depending on stage and tumor type. Regardless of disease stage, over 90% of all newly diagnosed cases of testicular cancer will be cured.
Balance of Benefits and Harms	Screening by self-examination or clinician examination is unlikely to offer meaningful health benefits, given the very low incidence and high cure rate of even advanced testicular cancer. Potential harms include false-positive results, anxiety, and harms from diagnostic tests or procedures.
Other Relevant USPSTF Recommendations	Recommendations on screening for other types of cancer can be found at http://www.uspreventiveservicestaskforce.org.

For a summary of the evidence systematically reviewed in making these recommendations, the full recommendation statement, and supporting documents, please go to http://www.uspreventiveservicestaskforce.org.

Tobacco Use in Adults

Title	Counseling and Interventions to Prevent Tobacco Use and Tobacco-Caused Disease in Adults and Pregnant Women	
Population	Adults age ≥ 18 years	Pregnant women of any age
Recommendation	Ask about tobacco use. Provide tobacco cessation interventions to those who use tobacco products. Grade: A	Ask about tobacco use. Provide augmented pregnancy-tailored counseling for women who smoke. Grade: A
Counseling	The "5-A" framework provides a useful counseling strategy: 1. **Ask** about tobacco use. 2. **Advise** to quit through clear personalized messages. 3. **Assess** willingness to quit. 4. **Assist** to quit. 5. **Arrange** follow-up and support. Intensity of counseling matters: brief one-time counseling works; however, longer sessions or multiple sessions are more effective. Telephone counseling "quit lines" also improve cessation rates.	
Pharmacotherapy	Combination therapy with counseling and medications is more effective than either component alone. FDA-approved pharmacotherapy includes nicotine replacement therapy, sustained-release bupropion, and varenicline.	The USPSTF found inadequate evidence to evaluate the safety or efficacy of pharmacotherapy during pregnancy.
Implementation	Successful implementation strategies for primary care practice include: • Instituting a tobacco user identification system. • Promoting clinician intervention through education, resources, and feedback. • Dedicating staff to provide treatment, and assessing the delivery of treatment in staff performance evaluations.	
Other Relevant USPSTF Recommendations	Recommendations on other behavioral counseling topics are available at http://www.uspreventiveservicestaskforce.org.	

Abbreviations: FDA = U.S. Food and Drug Administration; USPSTF = U.S. Preventive Services Task Force

For a summary of the evidence systematically reviewed in making these recommendations, the full recommendation statement, and supporting documents, please go to http://www.uspreventiveservicestaskforce.org.

61

Vitamin D and Calcium Supplementation to Prevent Fractures

Title	Vitamin D and Calcium Supplementation to Prevent Fractures in Adults		
Population	Men or premenopausal women	Community-dwelling postmenopausal women at doses of >400 IU of vitamin D_3 and >1,000 mg of calcium	Community-dwelling postmenopausal women at doses of ≤400 IU of vitamin D_3 and ≤1,000 mg of calcium
Recommendation	No recommendation. Grade: I (Insufficient Evidence)	No recommendation. Grade: I (Insufficient Evidence)	Do not supplement. Grade: D recommendation
Preventive Medications	Appropriate intake of vitamin D and calcium are essential to overall health. However, there is inadequate evidence to determine the effect of combined vitamin D and calcium supplementation on the incidence of fractures in men or premenopausal women. There is adequate evidence that daily supplementation with 400 IU of vitamin D_3 and 1,000 mg of calcium has no effect on the incidence of fractures in postmenopausal women. There is inadequate evidence regarding the effect of higher doses of combined vitamin D and calcium supplementation on fracture incidence in community-dwelling postmenopausal women.		
Balance of Benefits and Harms	Evidence is lacking regarding the benefit of daily vitamin D and calcium supplementation for the primary prevention of fractures, and the balance of benefits and harms cannot be determined.	Evidence is lacking regarding the benefit of daily supplementation with >400 IU of vitamin D_3 and >1,000 mg of calcium for the primary prevention of fractures in postmenopausal women, and the balance of benefits and harms cannot be determined.	Daily supplementation with ≤400 IU of vitamin D_3 and ≤1,000 mg of calcium has no net benefit for the primary prevention of fractures.
Other Relevant USPSTF Recommendations	The USPSTF has made recommendations on screening for osteoporosis and vitamin D supplementation to prevent falls in community-dwelling older adults. These recommendations are available at http://www.uspreventiveservicestaskforce.org/.		

For a summary of the evidence systematically reviewed in making this recommendation, the full recommendation statement, and supporting documents, please go to http://www.uspreventiveservicestaskforce.org/.

Vitamin Supplementation to Prevent Cardiovascular Disease and Cancer

Title	Vitamin, Mineral, and Multivitamin Supplements for the Primary Prevention of Cardiovascular Disease and Cancer	
Population	Healthy adults without special nutritional needs. This recommendation does not apply to children, women who are pregnant or may become pregnant, or persons who are chronically ill or hospitalized or have a known nutritional deficiency.	
Recommendation	Multivitamins: No recommendation. Grade: I statement	Single- or paired-nutrient supplements: No recommendation. Grade: I statement	β-carotene or vitamin E: Do not recommend. Grade: D

Preventive Medications	Evidence on supplementation with multivitamins to reduce the risk for cardiovascular disease or cancer is inadequate, as is the evidence on supplementation with individual vitamins, minerals, or functional pairs. Supplementation with β-carotene or vitamin E does not reduce the risk for cardiovascular disease or cancer.
Balance of Benefits and Harms	The evidence is insufficient to determine the balance of benefits and harms of supplementation with multivitamins for the prevention of cardiovascular disease or cancer. The evidence is insufficient to determine the balance of benefits and harms of supplementation with single or paired nutrients for the prevention of cardiovascular disease or cancer. There is no net benefit of supplementation with vitamin E or β-carotene for the prevention of cardiovascular disease or cancer.
Other Relevant USPSTF Recommendations	The USPSTF has made several recommendations on the prevention of cardiovascular disease and cancer, including recommendations for smoking cessation; screening for lipid disorders, hypertension, diabetes, and cancer; obesity screening and counseling; and aspirin use. These recommendations are available at http://www.uspreventiveservicestaskforce.org/.

For a summary of the evidence systematically reviewed in making this recommendation, the full recommendation statement, and supporting documents, please go to http://www.uspreventiveservicestaskforce.org/.

Clinical Summaries of Recommendations for Children and Adolescents

All clinical summaries in this Guide are abridged recommendations. To see the full recommendation statements and recommendations published after March 2014, go to www.USPreventiveServicesTaskForce.org.

—

Blood Lead Levels in Children and Pregnant Women

Title	Screening for Elevated Blood Lead Levels in Children and Pregnant Women		
Population	Asymptomatic children ages 1 to 5 years who are at increased risk	Asymptomatic children ages 1 to 5 years who are at average risk	Asymptomatic pregnant women
Recommendation	No recommendation. Grade: I (Insufficient Evidence)	Do not screen for elevated blood lead levels. Grade: D	Do not screen for elevated blood lead levels. Grade: D
Risk Assessment	Children younger than age 5 years are at greater risk for elevated blood lead levels and lead toxicity because of increased hand-to-mouth activity, increased lead absorption from the gastrointestinal tract, and the greater vulnerability of the developing central nervous system. Risk factors for increased blood lead levels in children and adults include: minority race/ethnicity; urban residence; low income; low educational attainment; older (pre-1950) housing; recent or ongoing home renovation or remodeling; pica; use of ethnic remedies, certain cosmetics, and exposure to lead-glazed pottery; occupational exposure; and recent immigration. Additional risk factors for pregnant women include alcohol use and smoking.		
Screening Tests	Venous sampling accurately detects elevated blood lead levels. Screening questionnaires may be of value in identifying children at risk for elevated blood lead levels, but should be tailored for and validated in specific communities for clinical use.		
Interventions	Treatment options for elevated blood lead levels include residential lead hazard-control efforts (i.e., counseling and education, dust or paint removal, and soil abatement), chelation, and nutritional interventions. Community-based interventions for the prevention of lead exposure are likely to be more effective, and may be more cost-effective, than office-based screening, treatment, and counseling. Relocating children who do not yet have elevated blood lead levels but who live in settings with high lead exposure may be especially helpful.		
Balance of Benefits and Harms	There is not enough evidence to assess the balance between the potential benefits and harms of routine screening for elevated blood lead levels in children at increased risk.	Given the significant potential harms of treatment and residential lead hazard abatement, and no evidence of treatment benefit, the harms of screening for elevated blood lead levels in children at average risk outweigh the benefits.	Given the significant potential harms of treatment and residential lead hazard abatement, and no evidence of treatment benefit, the harms of screening for elevated blood lead levels in asymptomatic pregnant women outweigh the benefits.

For a summary of the evidence systematically reviewed in making this recommendation, the full recommendation statement, and supporting documents, please go to http://www.uspreventiveservicestaskforce.org/.

67

Child Maltreatment

Title	Primary Care Interventions to Prevent Child Maltreatment
Population	Children and adolescents aged 0 to 18 years without signs or symptoms of maltreatment
Recommendation	**No recommendation.** **Grade: I (Insufficient Evidence)**
Risk Assessment	There are numerous risk factors associated with child maltreatment, including but not limited to: • Young, single, or nonbiological parents • Parental lack of understanding of childrenís needs, child development, or parenting skills • Poor parent–child relationships/negative interactions • Parental thoughts or emotions that support maltreatment behaviors • Family dysfunction or violence • Parental history of abuse or neglect in family of origin • Substance abuse within the family • Social isolation, poverty, or other socioeconomic disadvantages • Parental stress and distress
Interventions	Although the evidence is insufficient to recommend specific preventive interventions, most child maltreatment prevention programs focus on home visitation. Home visitation programs usually comprise a combination of services provided by a nurse or paraprofessional in the family's home on a regularly scheduled basis; most programs are targeted to families with young children and often begin in the prenatal or postnatal period.
Balance of Benefits and Harms	The evidence on interventions in primary care to prevent child maltreatment among children without signs or symptoms of maltreatment is insufficient, and the balance of benefits and harms cannot be determined.
Other Relevant USPSTF Recommendations	The USPSTF has made recommendations on screening for intimate partner violence and abuse of elderly and vulnerable adults. These recommendations are available at http://www.uspreventiveservicestaskforce.org/.

For a summary of the evidence systematically reviewed in making this recommendation, the full recommendation statement, and supporting documents, please go to http://www.uspreventiveservicestaskforce.org/.

Congenital Hypothyroidism

Title	Screening for Congenital Hypothyroidism
Population	All newborn infants[1]
Recommendation	**Screen for congenital hypothyroidism.** **Grade: A**

Screening Tests	Two methods of screening are used most frequently in the United States: • Primary TSH with backup T4. • Primary T4 with backup TSH. Screening for congenital hypothyroidism (CH) is mandated in all 50 states and the District of Columbia. Clinicians should become familiar with the tests used in their area and the limitations of the screening strategies employed.
Timing of Screening	Infants should be tested between 2 and 4 days of age. Infants discharged from hospitals before 48 hours of life should be tested immediately before discharge. Specimens obtained in the first 24-48 hours of age may be falsely elevated for TSH regardless of the screening method used.
Suggestions for Practice	Infants with abnormal screens should receive confirmatory testing and begin appropriate treatment with thyroid hormone replacement within 2 weeks after birth. Children with positive confirmatory testing in whom no permanent cause of CH is found should undergo a 30-day trial of reduced or discontinued thyroid hormone replacement therapy to determine if the hypothyroidism is permanent or transient. This trial of reduced or discontinued therapy should take place at some time after the child reaches 3 years of age.
Other Relevant Recommendations from the USPSTF	Additional USPSTF recommendations regarding screening tests for newborns can be accessed at: http://www.uspreventiveservicestaskforce.org/recommendations.htm#pediatric

[1]This recommendation applies to all infants born in the U.S. Premature, very low birth weight and ill infants may benefit from additional screening. These conditions are associated with decreased sensitivity and specificity of screening tests.

For a summary of the evidence systematically reviewed in making these recommendations, the full recommendation statement, and supporting documents, please go to http://www.uspreventiveservicestaskforce.org.

Developmental Dysplasia of the Hip

Title	Screening for Developmental Dysplasia of the Hip
Population	Infants who do not have obvious hip dislocations or other abnormalities evident without screening
Recommendation	No recommendation. Grade: I (Insufficient Evidence)

Risk Assessment	Risk factors for developmental dysplasia of the hip include female sex, family history, breech positioning, and in utero postural deformities. However, the majority of cases of developmental dysplasia of the hip have no identifiable risk factors.
Screening Tests	Screening tests for developmental dysplasia of the hip have limited accuracy. The most common methods of screening are serial physical examinations of the hip and lower extremities, using the Barlow and Ortolani procedures, and ultrasonography.
Interventions	Treatments for developmental dysplasia of the hip include both nonsurgical and surgical options. Nonsurgical treatment with abduction devices is used as early treatment and includes the commonly prescribed Pavlik method. Surgical intervention is used when the dysplasia is severe or diagnosed late, or after an unsuccessful trial of nonsurgical treatment. Avascular necrosis of the hip is the most common and most severe potential harm of both surgical and nonsurgical interventions, and can result in growth arrest of the hip and eventual joint destruction, with significant disability.
Balance of Benefits and Harms	The USPSTF was unable to assess the balance of benefits and harms of screening for developmental dysplasia of the hip due to insufficient evidence. There are concerns about the potential harms associated with treatment of infants identified by routine screening.
Other Relevant USPSTF Recommendations	The USPSTF has made recommendations on screening for hyperbilirubinemia, phenylketonuria, sickle cell disease, congenital hypothyroidism, and hearing loss in newborns. These recommendations are available at http://www.uspreventiveservicestaskforce.org/.

For a summary of the evidence systematically reviewed in making this recommendation, the full recommendation statement, and supporting documents, please go to http://www.uspreventiveservicestaskforce.org/.

Gonococcal Ophthalmia Neonatorum

Title	Ocular Prophylaxis for Gonococcal Ophthalmia Neonatorum
Population	All newborn infants
Recommendation	**Provide prophylactic ocular topical medication for the prevention of gonococcal ophthalmia neonatorum.** **Grade: A**

Risk Assessment	All newborns should receive prophylaxis. However, some newborns are at increased risk, including those with a maternal history of no prenatal care, sexually transmitted infections, or substance abuse.
Preventive Interventions	Preventive medications include 0.5% erythromycin ophthalmic ointment, 1.0% solution of silver nitrate, and 1.0% tetracycline ointment. All are considered equally effective; however, the latter two are no longer available in the United States.
Timing of Intervention	Within 24 hours after birth.
Other Relevant USPSTF Recommendations	Several recommendations on screening and counseling for infectious diseases and perinatal care can be found at: http://www.uspreventiveservicestaskforce.org.

For a summary of the evidence systematically reviewed in making these recommendations, the full recommendation statement, and supporting documents, please go to http://www.uspreventiveservicestaskforce.org.

Hearing Loss (Newborns)

Title	Universal Screening for Hearing Loss in Newborns
Population	All newborn infants
Recommendation	Screen for hearing loss in all newborn infants. Grade: B
Risk Assessment	The prevalence of hearing loss in newborn infants with specific risk indicators is 10 to 20 times higher than in the general population of newborns. Risk indicators associated with permanent bilateral congenital hearing loss include: • Neonatal intensive care unit admission for 2 or more days. • Family history of hereditary childhood sensorineural hearing loss. • Craniofacial abnormalities. • Certain congenital syndromes and infections. Approximately 50% of newborns with permanent bilateral congenital hearing loss do not have any known risk indicators.
Screening Tests	Screening programs should be conducted using a one-step or two-step validated protocol. A frequently-used 2-step screening process involves otoacoustic emissions followed by auditory brain stem response in newborns who fail the first test. Infants with positive screening tests should receive appropriate audiologic evaluation and follow-up after discharge. Procedures for screening and follow-up should be in place for newborns delivered at home, birthing centers, or hospitals without hearing screening facilities.
Timing of Screening	All infants should have hearing screening before one month of age. Infants who do not pass the newborn screening should undergo audiologic and medical evaluation before 3 months of age.
Treatment	Early intervention services for hearing-impaired infants should meet the individualized needs of the infant and family, including acquisition of communication competence, social skills, emotional well-being, and positive self-esteem. Early intervention comprises evaluation for amplification or sensory devices, surgical and medical evaluation, and communication assessment and therapy. Cochlear implants are usually considered for children with severe-to-profound hearing loss only after inadequate response to hearing aids.
Other Relevant USPSTF Recommendations	Additional USPSTF recommendations regarding screening tests for newborns can be accessed at http://www.uspreventiveservicestaskforce.org/recommendations.htm#pediatric.

For a summary of the evidence systematically reviewed in making these recommendations, the full recommendation statement, and supporting documents, please go to http://www.uspreventiveservicestaskforce.org.

High Blood Pressure (Children)

Title	Screening for Primary Hypertension in Children and Adolescents
Population	Children and adolescents without symptoms of hypertension
Recommendation	No recommendation. Grade: I (Insufficient Evidence)

Risk Assessment	The strongest risk factor for primary hypertension in children is elevated body mass index. Other risk factors include low birthweight, male sex, ethnicity, and a family history of hypertension.
Screening Tests	Blood pressure screening with sphygmomanometry in the clinical setting may identify children and adolescents with hypertension with reasonable sensitivity; however, false-positive results may occur with normalization of subsequent blood pressure measurements.
Treatment	Stage 1 hypertension in children is treated with lifestyle and pharmacological interventions; medications are not recommended as first-line therapy.
Balance of Benefits and Harms	The USPSTF found inadequate evidence on the diagnostic accuracy of screening for primary hypertension. The USPSTF also found inadequate evidence on the effectiveness of treatment and the harms of screening or treatment. Therefore, the USPSTF cannot determine the balance of benefits and harms of screening for hypertension in children and adolescents.
Other Relevant USPSTF Recommendations	The USPSTF has made recommendations on screening for lipid disorders in children and adolescents. These recommendations are available at http://www.uspreventiveservicestaskforce.org/.

For a summary of the evidence systematically reviewed in making this recommendation, the full recommendation statement, and supporting documents, please go to http://www.uspreventiveservicestaskforce.org/.

Hyperbilirubinemia in Infants

Title	Screening of Infants for Hyperbilirubinemia to Prevent Chronic Bilirubin Encephalopathy
Population	Healthy newborn infants ≥35 weeks' gestational age
Recommendation	No recommendation. Grade: I (Insufficient Evidence)

Risk Assessment	Risk factors for hyperbilirubinemia include family history of neonatal jaundice, exclusive breastfeeding, bruising, cephalohematoma, ethnicity (Asian, black), maternal age >25 years, male gender, G6PD deficiency, and gestational age <36 weeks. The specific contribution of these risk factors to chronic bilirubin encephalopathy in healthy children is not well understood.
Importance	Chronic bilirubin encephalopathy is a rare but devastating condition. Not all children with chronic bilirubin encephalopathy have a history of hyperbilirubinemia.
Balance of Benefits and Harms	Evidence about the benefits and harms of screening is lacking. Therefore, the USPSTF could not determine the balance of benefits and harms of screening newborns for hyperbilirubinemia to prevent chronic bilirubin encephalopathy.
Considerations for Practice	In deciding whether to screen, clinicians should consider the following: • **Potential preventable burden.** Bilirubin encephalopathy is a relatively rare disorder. Hyperbilirubinemia alone does not account for the neurologic condition of chronic bilirubin encephalopathy. There is no known screening test that will reliably identify all infants at risk of developing chronic bilirubin encephalopathy. • **Potential harms.** Potential harms of screening are unmeasured but may be important. Evidence about the potential harms of phototherapy is lacking. Harms of treatment by exchange transfusion may include apnea, bradycardia, cyanosis, vasospasm, thrombosis, necrotizing enterocolitis, and, rarely, death. • **Current practice.** Universal screening is widespread in the United States.
Screening Tests	Screening may consist of risk-factor assessment, measurement of bilirubin level either in serum or by transcutaneous estimation, or a combination of methods.
Interventions	Phototherapy is commonly used to treat hyperbilirubinemia. Exchange transfusion is used to treat extreme hyperbilirubinemia.
Relevant USPSTF Recommendations	USPSTF recommendations on screening newborns for hearing loss, congenital hypothyroidism, hemoglobinopathies, and phenylketonuria (PKU) can be found at http://www.uspreventiveservicestaskforce.org.

For a summary of the evidence systematically reviewed in making these recommendations, the full recommendation statement, and supporting documents, please go to http://www.uspreventiveservicestaskforce.org.

Illicit and Prescription Drug Use in Children and Adolescents

Title	Primary Care Behavioral Interventions to Reduce Illicit Drug and Nonmedical Pharmaceutical Use in Children and Adolescents
Population	Children and adolescents younger than age 18 years who have not already been diagnosed with a substance use disorder
Recommendation	No recommendation. **Grade: I statement**

Behavioral Interventions	While the evidence is insufficient to recommend specific interventions in the primary care setting, those that have been studied include face-to-face counseling, videos, print materials, and interactive computer-based tools. Studies on these interventions were limited and findings on whether interventions significantly improved health outcomes were inconsistent.
Balance of Benefits and Harms	The evidence regarding primary care–based behavioral interventions to prevent or reduce illicit drug and nonmedical pharmaceutical use in children and adolescents is insufficient, and the balance of benefits and harms cannot be determined.
Other Relevant USPSTF Recommendations	The USPSTF has made recommendations on screening for and interventions to decrease the unhealthy use of other substances, including alcohol and tobacco. These recommendations are available at www.uspreventiveservicestaskforce.org.

For a summary of the evidence systematically reviewed in making this recommendation, the full recommendation statement, and supporting documents, please go to http://www.uspreventiveservicestaskforce.org/.

Iron Deficiency Anemia (Screening)

Title	Part I: Screening for Iron Deficiency Anemia in Children and Pregnant Women	
Population	Asymptomatic children ages 6 to 12 months	Asymptomatic pregnant women
Recommendation	No recommendation. Grade: I (Insufficient Evidence)	Screen for iron deficiency anemia. Grade: B
Risk Assessment	Individuals considered to be at high risk for iron deficiency include adult women, recent immigrants, and, among adolescent females, fad dieters, as well as those who are obese. Premature and low birth weight infants are also at increased risk for iron deficiency.	
Screening Tests	Serum hemoglobin or hematocrit is the primary screening test for identifying anemia. Hemoglobin is sensitive for iron deficiency anemia; however, it is not sensitive for iron deficiency because mild deficiency states may not affect hemoglobin levels. Potential harms of screening include false-positive results, anxiety, and cost.	
Interventions	Iron deficiency anemia is usually treated with oral iron preparations. The likelihood that iron deficiency anemia identified by screening will respond to treatment is unclear, because many families do not adhere to treatment and because the rate of spontaneous resolution is high.	
Balance of Benefits and Harms	The USPSTF was unable to determine the balance between the benefits and harms of routine screening for iron deficiency anemia in asymptomatic children ages 6 to 12 months.	The benefits of routine screening for iron deficiency anemia in asymptomatic pregnant women outweigh the potential harms.
Other Relevant USPSTF Recommendations	The USPSTF has also made recommendations on screening for blood lead levels in children and pregnant women. These recommendations are available at http://www.uspreventiveservicestaskforce.org/.	

For a summary of the evidence systematically reviewed in making this recommendation, the full recommendation statement, and supporting documents, please go to http://www.uspreventiveservicestaskforce.org/.

Iron Deficiency Anemia (Supplementation)

	Part II: Iron Supplementation for Children and Pregnant Women		
Title			
Population	Asymptomatic children ages 6 to 12 months who are at increased risk for iron deficiency anemia	Asymptomatic children ages 6 to 12 months who are at average risk for iron deficiency anemia	Pregnant women who are not anemic
Recommendation	Provide routine iron supplementation. **Grade: B**	No recommendation. **Grade: I (Insufficient Evidence)**	No recommendation. **Grade: I (Insufficient Evidence)**
Risk Assessment	A validated risk assessment tool to guide primary care physicians in identifying individuals who would benefit from iron supplementation has not been developed.		
Preventive Medication	Iron supplementation, such as iron-fortified formula or iron supplements, may improve neurodevelopmental outcomes in children at increased risk for iron deficiency anemia. There is poor evidence that it improves neurodevelopmental or health outcomes in other populations. Oral iron supplementation increases the risk for unintentional overdose and gastrointestinal symptoms. Given appropriate protection against overdose, these harms are small.		
Balance of Benefits and Harms	The moderate benefits of iron supplementation in asymptomatic children ages 6 to 12 months who are at increased risk for iron deficiency anemia outweigh the potential harms.	The USPSTF was unable to determine the balance between the benefits and harms of iron supplementation in children ages 6 to 12 months who are at average risk for iron deficiency anemia.	The USPSTF was unable to determine the balance between the benefits and harms of iron supplementation in non-anemic pregnant women.
Other Relevant USPSTF Recommendations	The USPSTF has also made recommendations on folic acid supplementation in women planning or capable of pregnancy and vitamin D supplementation to prevent cancer and fractures. These recommendations are available at http://www.uspreventiveservicestaskforce.org/.		

For a summary of the evidence systematically reviewed in making this recommendation, the full recommendation statement, and supporting documents, please go to http://www.uspreventiveservicestaskforce.org/.

Lipid Disorders in Children

Title	Screening for Lipid Disorders in Children
Population	Asymptomatic infants, children, adolescents, and young adults (age 20 years or younger)
Recommendation	No recommendation. Grade: I (Insufficient Evidence)

Risk Assessment	Risk factors for dyslipidemia include overweight, diabetes, and a family history of common familial dyslipidemias (e.g., familial hypercholesterolemia).
Screening Tests	Serum lipid (total cholesterol, high-density and low-density lipoprotein cholesterol) levels are accurate screening tests for childhood dyslipidemia, although many children with multifactorial types of dyslipidemia will have normal lipid levels in adulthood. The use of family history as a screening tool for dyslipidemia has variable accuracy, largely because definitions of a positive family history and lipid threshold values vary substantially.
Interventions	The effectiveness of treatment interventions (diet, exercise, lipid-lowering agents) in improving health outcomes in children with dyslipidemia (including multifactorial dyslipidemia) remains a critical research gap. Potential harms of screening may include labeling of children whose dyslipidemia would not persist into adulthood or cause health problems. Adverse effects from lipid-lowering medications and low-fat diets, including potential long-term harms, have been inadequately evaluated in children.
Balance of Benefits and Harms	The USPSTF was unable to determine the balance between the potential benefits and harms of routinely screening children and adolescents for dyslipidemia.
Other Relevant USPSTF Recommendations	The USPSTF has made recommendations on high blood pressure and obesity in children and adolescents. These recommendations are available at http://www.uspreventiveservicestaskforce.org/.

For a summary of the evidence systematically reviewed in making this recommendation, the full recommendation statement, and supporting documents, please go to http://www.uspreventiveservicestaskforce.org/.

78

Major Depressive Disorder in Children and Adolescents

Title	Screening and Treatment for Major Depressive Disorder in Children and Adolescents	
Population	Adolescents (12-18 years)	Children (7-11 years)
Recommendation	Screen when systems for diagnosis, treatment, and followup are in place. Grade: B	No Recommendation Grade: I (Insufficient Evidence)

Risk Assessment	Risk factors for major depressive disorder (MDD) include parental depression, having comorbid mental health or chronic medical conditions, and having experienced a major negative life event.	
Screening Tests	The following screening tests have been shown to do well in teens in primary care settings: • Patient Health Questionnaire for Adolescents (PHQ-A). • Beck Depression Inventory-Primary Care Version (BDI-PC).	Screening instruments perform less well in younger children.
Treatments	Among pharmacotherapies fluoxetine, a selective serotonin reuptake inhibitor (SSRI), has been found efficacious. However, because of risk of suicidality, SSRIs should be considered only if clinical monitoring is possible. Various modes of psychotherapy, and pharmacotherapy combined with psychotherapy, have been found efficacious.	Evidence on the balance of benefits and harms of treatment of younger children is insufficient for a recommendation.

For a summary of the evidence systematically reviewed in making these recommendations, the full recommendation statement, and supporting documents, please go to http://www.uspreventiveservicestaskforce.org.

Obesity in Children and Adolescents

Title	Screening for Obesity in Children and Adolescents
Population	Children and adolescents 6 to 18 years of age
Recommendation	**Screen children aged 6 years and older for obesity.** **Offer or refer for intensive counseling and behavioral interventions.** Grade: B

Screening Tests	BMI is calculated from the weight in kilograms divided by the square of the height in meters. Height and weight, from which BMI is calculated, are routinely measured during health maintenance visits. BMI percentile can be plotted on a chart or obtained from online calculators. Overweight = age- and gender-specific BMI at ≥85th to 94th percentile Obesity = age- and gender-specific BMI at ≥95th percentile
Timing of Screening	No evidence was found on appropriate screening intervals.
Interventions	Refer patients to comprehensive moderate- to high-intensity programs that include dietary, physical activity, and behavioral counseling components.
Balance of Benefits and Harms	Moderate- to high-intensity programs were found to yield modest weight changes. Limited evidence suggests that these improvements can be sustained over the year after treatment. Harms of screening were judged to be minimal.
Other Relevant USPSTF Recommendations	Recommendations on other pediatric and behavioral counseling topics can be found at http://www.uspreventiveservicestaskforce.org.

For a summary of the evidence systematically reviewed in making these recommendations, the full recommendation statement, and supporting documents, please go to http://www.uspreventiveservicestaskforce.org.

Phenylketonuria (PKU)

Title	Screening for Phenylketonuria
Population	All newborn infants
Recommendation	Screen for Phenykeltonuria (PKU). Grade: A

Screening Tests	Screening for PKU is mandated in all 50 states. Methods of screening vary. Three main methods are used to screen for PKU in the United States: 1. Guthrie Bacterial Inhibition Assay (BIA) 2. Automated fluorometric assay 3. Tandem mass spectrometry
Timing of Screening	Infants who are tested within the first 24 hours after birth should receive a repeat screening test by 2 weeks of age. Optimal timing of screening for premature infants and infants with illnesses is at or near 7 days of age, but in all cases before discharge from the newborn nursery.
Treatment	It is essential that phenylalanine restrictions be instituted shortly after birth to prevent the neurodevelopmental effects of PKU.
Other Relevant USPSTF Recommendations	Additional USPSTF recommendations regarding screening tests for newborns can be accessed at: http://www.uspreventiveservicestaskforce.org/recommendations.htm#pediatric

For a summary of the evidence systematically reviewed in making these recommendations, the full recommendation statement, and supporting documents, please go to http://www.uspreventiveservicestaskforce.org.

Sickle Cell Disease

Title	Screening for Sickle Cell Disease in Newborns
Population	All newborn infants
Recommendation	Screen for sickle cell disease. Grade: A

Screening Tests	Screening for sickle cell disease in newborns is mandated in all 50 states and the District of Columbia. In most states, one of these tests is used for the initial screening: • Thin-layer isoelectric focusing (IEF). • High performance liquid chromatography (HPLC). Both IEF and HPLC have extremely high sensitivity and specificity for sickle cell anemia.
Timing of Screening	All newborns should undergo screening regardless of birth setting. Birth attendants should make arrangements for samples to be obtained. The first clinician to see the infant at an office visit should verify screening results. Confirmatory testing should occur no later than 2 months of age.
Treatment	Infants with sickle cell anemia should receive: • Prophylactic penicillin starting by age 2 months. • Pneumococcal immunizations at recommended intervals.
Other Relevant USPSTF Recommendations	Additional USPSTF recommendations regarding screening tests for newborns can be accessed at http://www.uspreventiveservicestaskforce.org/recommendations.htm#vision.

For a summary of the evidence systematically reviewed in making these recommendations, the full recommendation statement, and supporting documents, please go to http://www.uspreventiveservicestaskforce.org.

Speech and Language Delay

Title	Screening for Speech and Language Delay in Preschool Children
Population	Children ages 5 years and younger who have not already been identified as at increased risk for speech and language delays
Recommendation	No recommendation. Grade: I (Insufficient Evidence)

Risk Assessment	The most consistently reported risk factors include a family history of speech and language delay, male sex, and perinatal factors, such as prematurity and low birth-weight. Other risk factors reported less consistently include levels of parental education, specific childhood illnesses, birth order, and larger family size.
Screening Tests	There is insufficient evidence that brief, formal screening instruments that are suitable for use in primary care for assessing speech and language development can accurately identify children who would benefit from further evaluation and intervention.
Balance of Benefits and Harms	The USPSTF could not determine the balance of benefits and harms of using brief, formal screening instruments to screen for speech and language delay in the primary care setting.
Other Relevant USPSTF Recommendations	The USPSTF has also made recommendations on screening for hearing loss in newborns and vision impairment in children ages 1 to 5 years. These recommendations are available at http://www.uspreventiveservicestaskforce.org/.

For a summary of the evidence systematically reviewed in making this recommendation, the full recommendation statement, and supporting documents, please go to http://www.uspreventiveservicestaskforce.org/.

Tobacco Use in Children and Adolescents

Title	Primary Care Interventions to Prevent Tobacco Use in Children and Adolescents
Population	School-aged children and adolescents
Recommendation	Provide interventions to prevent initiation of tobacco use. Grade: B

Risk Assessment	The strongest factors associated with smoking initiation in children and adolescents are parental smoking and parental nicotine dependence. Other factors include low levels of parental monitoring, easy access to cigarettes, perception that peers smoke, and exposure to tobacco promotions.
Behavioral Counseling Interventions	Behavioral counseling interventions, such as face-to-face or phone interaction with a health care provider, print materials, and computer applications, can reduce the risk for smoking initiation in school-aged children and adolescents. The type and intensity of effective behavioral interventions substantially varies.
Balance of Benefits and Harms	There is a moderate net benefit to providing primary care interventions to prevent tobacco use in school-aged children and adolescents.
Other Relevant USPSTF Recommendations	The USPSTF has made recommendations on counseling and interventions to prevent tobacco use and tobacco-caused disease in adults and pregnant women. These recommendations are available at www.uspreventiveservicestaskforce.org/.

For a summary of the evidence systematically reviewed in making this recommendation, the full recommendation statement, and supporting documents, please go to http://www.uspreventiveservicestaskforce.org/.

Visual Impairment in Children Ages 1 to 5

Title	Screening for Visual Impairment in Children Ages 1 to 5	
Population	Children ages 3 to 5 years	Children younger than 3 years of age
Recommendation	Provide vision screening. Grade: B	No recommendation. Grade: I (Insufficient Evidence)
Screening Tests	Various screening tests are used in primary care to identify visual impairment in children, including: • Visual acuity test • Stereoacuity test • Cover-uncover test • Hirschberg light reflex test • Autorefraction • Photoscreening	
Timing of Screening	No evidence was found regarding appropriate screening intervals.	
Interventions	Primary treatment for amblyopia includes the use of corrective lenses, patching, or atropine therapy of the non-affected eye. Treatment may also consist of a combination of interventions.	
Balance of Benefits and Harms	There is adequate evidence that early treatment of amblyopia in children ages 3 to 5 years leads to improved visual outcomes. There is limited evidence on harms of screening, including psychosocial effects, in children ages 3 years and older. There is inadequate evidence that early treatment of amblyopia in children younger than 3 years of age leads to improved visual outcomes.	
Suggestions for Practice Regarding the I Statement	In deciding whether to refer children younger than 3 years of age for screening, clinicians should consider: • *Potential preventable burden:* screening later in the preschool years seems to be as effective as screening earlier • *Costs:* initial high costs associated with autorefractors and photoscreeners • *Current practice:* typical vision screening includes assessment of visual acuity, strabismus, and stereoacuity; children with positive findings should be referred for a comprehensive ophthalmologist exam	

For a summary of the evidence systematically reviewed in making these recommendations, the full recommendation statement, and supporting documents, please go to http://www.uspreventiveservicestaskforce.org.

Immunizations for Adults and Children

Immunizations for Adults and Children

The USPSTF recognizes the importance of immunizations in primary disease prevention. However, the USPSTF does not wish to duplicate the significant investment of resources made by others to review new evidence on immunizations in a timely fashion and make recommendations.

The Centers for Disease Control and Prevention's (CDC's) Advisory Committee on Immunization Practices (ACIP) publishes recommendations on immunizations for children and adults. The methods used by the ACIP to review evidence on immunizations may differ from the methods used by the USPTF.

For the ACIP's current recommendations on immunizations, please refer to the National Immunization Program Web site at www.cdc.gov/vaccines/recs/schedules/default.htm.

Topics in Progress

Each USPSTF recommendation goes through several stages of development. The review process takes into account input from the medical and research community, stakeholders, and the general public.

The length of time for the entire recommendation process varies depending on the amount and type of available evidence and the time required for compilation of data into a draft recommendation, public comment periods, consideration of comments, and in-depth review and discussions among USPSTF members.

The following topics are in review and are likely to be issued as drafts for public comment during 2014:

- Aspirin for the Prevention of Cardiovascular Disease
- Aspirin or NSAIDS for the Prevention of Colorectal Cancer, Preventive Medications
- Aspirin Use to Prevent Preeclampsia, Preventive Medications
- Chlamydial Infection, Screening
- Diabetes Mellitus, Screening
- Gonorrhea, Screening
- Healthy Diet and Physical Activity for Cardiovascular Disease Prevention in Adults at Risk, Counseling
- High Blood Pressure in Adults, Screening
- Iron Deficiency Anemia in Childhood and Pregnancy, Screening
- Major Depressive Disorder in Children and Adolescents, Screening
- Sexually Transmitted Infections, Counseling
- Thyroid Disease, Screening
- Vitamin D Deficiency, Screening

Recommendations on the following topics were published during the production of the *2014 Guide to Clinical Preventive Services* or are in review and are likely to be published as final recommendations during 2014:

- Abdominal Aortic Aneurysm, Screening
- Carotid Artery Stenosis, Screening
- Dental Caries Prevention in Children From Birth to Age 5 Years, Screening and Preventive Medications

- Hepatitis B Virus Infection in Nonpregnant Adolescents and Adults, Screening
- Suicide Risk, Screening

The following topics are in earlier stages of review and are likely to be issued as drafts or published as final recommendations sometime after 2014:

- Autism Spectrum Disorder in Young Children, Screening
- Breast Cancer, Screening
- Chronic Obstructive Pulmonary Disease, Screening
- Colorectal Cancer, Screening
- Depression in Adults and in Pregnant and Postpartum Women, Screening
- Impaired Visual Acuity in Older Adults, Screening
- Lipid Disorders in Adults, Screening
- Lipid Disorders in Children, Screening
- Skin Cancer, Screening
- Speech and Language Delay and Disorders in Children Age 5 Years or Younger, Screening
- Syphilis Infection, Screening
- Tobacco Cessation in Adults, Including Pregnant Women, Counseling

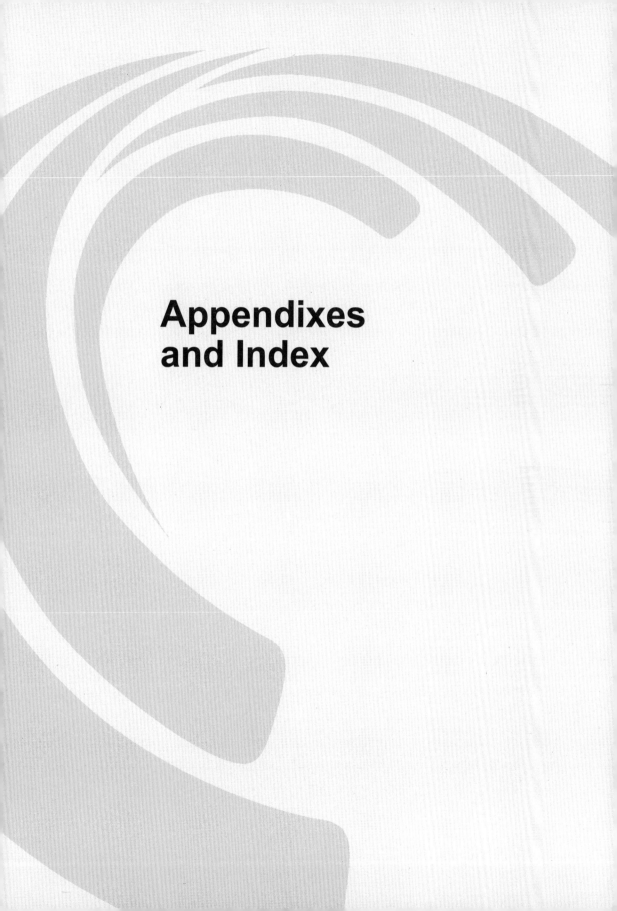

Appendixes
and Index

How the U.S. Preventive Services Task Force Grades Its Recommendations

The Task Force assigns each of its recommendations a letter grade (A, B, C, or D) or issues an I statement, based on the certainty of the evidence and on the balance of benefits and harms of the preventive service as displayed in the recommendation grid below. The USPSTF changed its grade definitions based on a change in methods in May 2007.

U.S. Preventive Services Task Force Recommendation Grid: Letter Grade of Recommendation or Statement of Insufficient Evidence Assessing Certainty and Magnitude of Net Benefit

Certainty of Net Benefit	Magnitude of Net Benefit			
	Substantial	Moderate	Small	Zero/negative
High	A	B	C	D
Moderate	B	B	C	D
Low	Insufficient			

Grade Definitions

What the Grades Mean and Suggestions for Practice

The USPSTF updated its definitions of the grades it assigns to recommendations and now includes "suggestions for practice" associated with each grade. The USPSTF has also defined levels of certainty regarding net benefit.

Grade	Definition	Suggestions for Practice
A	The USPSTF recommends the service. There is high certainty that the net benefit is substantial.	Offer or provide this service.
B	The USPSTF recommends the service. There is high certainty that the net benefit is moderate or there is moderate certainty that the net benefit is moderate to substantial.	Offer or provide this service.
C	The USPSTF recommends selectively offering or providing this service to individual patients based on professional judgment and patient preferences. There is at least moderate certainty that the net benefit is small.	Offer or provide this service for selected patients depending on individual circumstances.
D	The USPSTF recommends against the service. There is moderate or high certainty that the service has no net benefit or that the harms outweigh the benefits.	Discourage the use of this service.
I Statement	The USPSTF concludes that the current evidence is insufficient to assess the balance of benefits and harms of the service. Evidence is lacking, of poor quality, or conflicting, and the balance of benefits and harms cannot be determined.	Read the clinical considerations section of USPSTF Recommendation Statement. If the service is offered, patients should understand the uncertainty about the balance of benefits and harms.

Levels of Certainty Regarding Net Benefit

Level of Certainty*	Description
High	The available evidence usually includes consistent results from well-designed, well-conducted studies in representative primary care populations. These studies assess the effects of the preventive service on health outcomes. This conclusion is therefore unlikely to be strongly affected by the results of future studies.
Moderate	The available evidence is sufficient to determine the effects of the preventive service on health outcomes, but confidence in the estimate is constrained by such factors as: • The number, size, or quality of individual studies. • Inconsistency of findings across individual studies. • Limited generalizability of findings to routine primary care practice. • Lack of coherence in the chain of evidence. As more information becomes available, the magnitude or direction of the observed effect could change, and this change may be large enough to alter the conclusion.
Low	The available evidence is insufficient to assess effects on health outcomes. Evidence is insufficient because of: • The limited number or size of studies. • Important flaws in study design or methods. • Inconsistency of findings across individual studies. • Gaps in the chain of evidence. • Findings not generalizable to routine primary care practice. • Lack of information on important health outcomes. More information may allow estimation of effects on health outcomes.

* The USPSTF defines certainty as "likelihood that the USPSTF assessment of the net benefit of a preventive service is correct." The net benefit is defined as benefit minus harm of the preventive service as implemented in a general, primary care population. The USPSTF assigns a certainty level based on the nature of the overall evidence available to assess the net benefit of a preventive service.

Grade Definitions Prior to May 2007

The definitions below (of USPSTF grades and quality of evidence ratings) were in use prior to the update and apply to recommendations voted on by the USPSTF prior to May 2007.

A — Strongly Recommended: The USPSTF strongly recommends that clinicians provide [the service] to eligible patients. The USPSTF found good evidence that [the service] improves important health outcomes and concludes that benefits substantially outweigh harms.

B — Recommended: The USPSTF recommends that clinicians provide [the service] to eligible patients. The USPSTF found at least fair evidence that [the service] improves important health outcomes and concludes that benefits outweigh harms.

C — No Recommendation: The USPSTF makes no recommendation for or against routine provision of [the service]. The USPSTF found at least fair evidence that [the service] can improve health outcomes but concludes that the balance of benefits and harms is too close to justify a general recommendation.

D — Not Recommended: The USPSTF recommends against routinely providing [the service] to asymptomatic patients. The USPSTF found at least fair evidence that [the service] is ineffective or that harms outweigh benefits.

I — Insufficient Evidence to Make a Recommendation: The USPSTF concludes that the evidence is insufficient to recommend for or against routinely providing [the service]. Evidence that [the service] is effective is lacking, of poor quality, or conflicting and the balance of benefits and harms cannot be determined.

Quality of Evidence Prior to May 2007

The USPSTF grades the quality of the overall evidence for a service on a 3-point scale (good, fair, poor):

Good: Evidence includes consistent results from well-designed, well-conducted studies in representative populations that directly assess effects on health outcomes.

Fair: Evidence is sufficient to determine effects on health outcomes, but the strength of the evidence is limited by the number, quality, or consistency of the individual studies, generalizability to routine practice, or indirect nature of the evidence on health outcomes.

Poor: Evidence is insufficient to assess the effects on health outcomes because of limited number or power of studies, important flaws in their design or conduct, gaps in the chain of evidence, or lack of information on important health outcomes.

Appendix B

Members of the U.S. Preventive Services Task Force 2004-2014

Janet D. Allan, Ph.D., R.N., C.S., F.A.A.N.
School of Nursing
University of Maryland, Baltimore
Baltimore, MD

Linda Ciofu Baumann, Ph.D., R.N.
School of Nursing and School of
    Medicine & Public Health
University of Wisconsin
Madison, WI

Alfred O. Berg, M.D., M.P.H.
University of Washington
Seattle, WA

Kirsten Bibbins-Domingo, Ph.D., M.D.
San Francisco General Hospital
University of California,
San Francisco, CA

Adelita Gonzales Cantu, R.N., Ph.D.
University of Texas Health Science
    Center
San Antonio, TX

Ned Calonge, M.D., M.P.H.
Colorado Department of Public Health
    and Environment
Denver, CO

Susan J. Curry, Ph.D.
College of Public Health
University of Iowa
Iowa City, IA

Karina W. Davidson, Ph.D., M.A.Sc.
Center for Behavioral Cardiovascular
    Health
Columbia University Medical Center
New York, NY

Thomas G. DeWitt, M.D.
Department of Pediatrics
Children's Hospital Medical Center
Cincinnati, OH

Allen J. Dietrich, M.D.
Dartmouth Medical School
Hanover, NH

Mark Ebell, M.D., M.S.
The University of Georgia
Athens, GA

Glenn Flores, M.D.
University of Texas
Southwestern Medical Center and
    Children's Medical Center of Dallas
Dallas, TX

Paul S. Frame, M.D.
Tri-County Family Medicine
Cohocton, MY

Francisco A.R. García, M.D., M.P.H.
Pima County Department of Health
Tucson, AZ

Matthew W. Gillman, M.D., S.M.
Obesity Prevention Program
Harvard Medical School and Harvard
    Pilgrim Health Care Institute
Boston, MA

Leon Gordis, M.D., Dr.P.H.
Johns Hopkins Bloomberg School of
    Public Health
Baltimore, MD

Kimberly D. Gregory, M.D., M.P.H.
Cedars-Sinai Medical Center
Los Angeles, CA

David Grossman, M.D., M.P.H.
Center for Health Studies, Group
   Health Cooperative
University of Washington
Seattle, WA

Russell Harris, M.D., M.P.H.
University of North Carolina School
   of Medicine
Chapel Hill, NC

Jessica Herzstein, M.D., M.P.H.
Air Products
Allentown, PA

George Isham, M.D., M.S.
HealthPartners
Minneapolis, MN

Mark S. Johnson, M.D., M.P.H.
New Jersey Medical School
University of Medicine and Dentistry of
   New Jersey
Newark, NJ

Alex R. Kemper, M.D., M.P.H., M.S.
Pediatrics
Duke University Medical School
Durham, NC
Division of Children's Primary Care
Duke University
Durham, NC

Kenneth Kizer, M.D., M.P.H.
National Quality Forum
Washington, DC

Jonathan D. Klein, M.D., M.P.H.
University of Rochester
Rochester, NY

**Ann E. Kurth, Ph.D., R.N., M.S.N.,
M.P.H.**
College of Nursing and the Department
   of Population Health
Global Institute of Public Health
New York University
New York, NY

Michael L. LeFevre, M.D., M.S.P.H.
University of Missouri School of
   Medicine
Columbia, MO

Rosanne Leipzig, M.D., Ph.D.
Mount Sinai School of Medicine
New York, NY

**Carol Loveland-Cherry, Ph.D., R.N.,
F.A.A.N.**
School of Nursing
University of Michigan
Ann Arbor, MI

Lucy N. Marion, Ph.D., R.N.
School of Nursing
Medical College of Georgia
Augusta, GA

Joy Melnikow, M.D., M.P.H.
University of California Davis
Sacramento, CA

**Bernadette Melnyk, Ph.D., R.N.,
C.P.N.P./N.P.P.**
College of Nursing & Healthcare
   Innovation
Arizona State University
Phoenix, AZ

Virginia A. Moyer, M.D., M.P.H.
University of Texas Health Science
   Center
Houston, TX

**Wanda Nicholson, M.D., M.P.H.,
M.B.A.**
Johns Hopkins School of Medicine and
   Bloomberg School of Public Health
Baltimore, MD

Judith K. Ockene, Ph.D., M.Ed.
University of Massachusetts Medical
   School
Worcester, MA

Douglas K. Owens, M.D., M.S.
VA Palo Alto Health Care System
Freeman Spogli Institute for
    International Studies
Stanford University
Stanford, CA

Diana B. Petitti, M.D., M.P.H.
Fulton School of Engineering
Arizona State University
Tempe, AZ

William R. Phillips, M.D., M.P.H.
Family Medicine and Health Services
University of Washington
Seattle, WA

Maureen G. Phipps, M.D., M.P.H.
Department of Obstetrics and
Gynecology
Warren Alpert Medical School
Brown University, Providence, RI

Michael P. Pignone, M.D., M.P.H.
Division of General Internal Medicine
University of North Carolina
Chapel Hill, NC

Carolina Reyes, M.D.
University of Southern California,
    Los Angeles County/USC Medical
    Center
Los Angeles, CA

George F. Sawaya, M.D.
University of California, San Francisco
San Francisco, CA

J. Sanford (Sandy) Schwartz, M.D.
University of Pennsylvania School of
    Medicine and Wharton School
Philadelphia, PA

Albert L. Siu, M.D.
Mount Sinai Medical Center
New York, NY

Steven M. Teutsch, M.D., M.P.H.
Merck and Company, Inc.
West Point, PA

Timothy Wilt, M.D., M.P.H.
Minneapolis VA Medical Center
University of Minnesota
Minneapolis, MN

**Barbara P. Yawn, M.D., M.S.P.H.,
    M.Sc.**
Olmstead Medical Center
Rochester, MN

Appendix C

Acknowledgements

AHRQ Staff Supporting the USPSTF

Aileen Buckler, M.D., M.P.H.
Joel Boches
Joya Chowdhury, M.P.H.
Robert Cosby, Ph.D.
Jennifer Croswell, M.D., M.P.H.
Sandra K. Cummings
Farah Englert
Tina Fan, M.D., M.P.H.
Saeed Fatemi
Janice Genevro, Ph.D., M.S.W.
Margi Grady
Alison Hunt
William Hyde, M.L.S.
Kristie Kiser
Karen Lee, M.D., M.P.H.
Biff LeVee
Iris Mabry, M.D., M.P.H.
Corey Mackison, M.S.A.
Andrew Marshall
Robert McNellis, M.P.H., P.A.
David Meyers, M.D.
Tess Miller, Dr.P.H.
Emily Moser
Quyen Ngo-Metzger, M.D., M.P.H.
Lisa Nicolella
Linwood Norman, M.S.
Janine Payne, M.P.H.
Kathryn Ramage
Richard Ricciardi, Ph.D., N.P., F.A.A.N.P.
Randie Siegel, M.S.
Rachel Weinstein
Tracy Wolff, M.D., M.P.H.

Evidence-based Practice Centers Supporting the USPSTF 2014

Kaiser Permanente Research Affiliates Evidence-based Practice Center

Director, Evelyn P. Whitlock, M.D., M.P.H.

The Kaiser Permanente Research Affiliates EPC involves over 75 researchers from three integrated health care delivery systems: Kaiser Permanente, Group Health Research Institute, and HealthPartners Institute for Education and Research. The KPRA EPC is headquartered in Portland, Oregon, at the Kaiser Permanente Center for Health Research. To learn more about the KPRA EPC, please visit:

http://www.kpchr.org/research/public/resEPC.htm

Pacific Northwest Evidence-based Practice Center

Director, Roger Chou, M.D.

The Pacific Northwest EPC is housed in the Department of Medical Informatics & Clinical Epidemiology, at the Oregon Health and Science University School of Medicine, with partners at the University of Washington CHASE Alliance in Seattle, and Spectrum Research, Inc., in Tacoma, Washington. To learn more about the Pacific Northwest EPC, please visit:

http://www.ohsu.edu/xd/research/centers-institutes/evidence-based-practice-center/

RTI-UNC Evidence-based Practice Center

Director, Meena Viswanathan, Ph.D.

Co-Director, Dan Jonas, M.D., M.P.H.

RTI International, in collaboration with the five health professions schools and the Cecil G. Sheps Center for Health Services Research at the University of North Carolina at Chapel Hill, operates the RTI-UNC Evidence-based Practice Center. To learn more about the RTI-UNC EPC, please visit:

http://www.rti.org/page.cfm?objectid=4FA3323C-51CA-4DFE-A3E0246F90D5FA4B.

Vanderbilt Evidence-based Practice Center

Director, Melissa McPheeters, Ph.D., M.P.H.

Established in 2007, the Vanderbilt EPC is located in the Institute for Medicine and Public Health at Vanderbilt University. To learn more about the Vanderbilt EPC, please visit:

http://medicineandpublichealth.vanderbilt.edu/epc/.

Liaisons to the USPSTF

Primary care partners include:

- American Academy of Family Physicians (AAFP)
- American Academy of Nurse Practitioners (AANP)
- American Academy of Pediatrics (AAP)
- American Academy of Physician Assistants (AAPA)
- American Congress of Obstetricians and Gynecologists (ACOG)
- American College of Physicians (ACP)
- American College of Preventive Medicine (ACPM)
- American Osteopathic Association (AOA)
- National Association of Pediatric Nurse Practitioners (NAPNAP)

Policy, population, and quality improvement partners include:

- America's Health Insurance Plans (AHIP)
- American Medical Association
- National Committee for Quality Assurance (NCQA)
- AARP
- Canadian Task Force on Preventive Health Care (CTFPHC)
- Community Preventive Services Task Force (CPSTF)

Federal partners include:

- Centers for Disease Control and Prevention (CDC)
- Centers for Medicare & Medicaid Services (CMS)
- Department of Defense/Military Health System (DoD/MHS)
- U.S. Food and Drug Administration (FDA)
- Health Resources and Services Administration (HRSA)
- Indian Health Service (IHS)
- National Institutes of Health (NIH)
- Veteran's Health Administration (VHA)
- Substance Abuse & Mental Health Services Administration (SAMHSA)
- Office of the Assistant Secretary for Planning and Evaluation (ASPE)
- Office of Disease Prevention and Health Promotion (ODPHP)
- Office of the Surgeon General

Appendix D

About the U.S. Preventive Services Task Force

Overview

Created in 1984, the U.S. Preventive Services Task Force (USPSTF) is an independent group of national experts in prevention and evidence-based medicine that works to improve the health of all Americans by making evidence-based recommendations about clinical preventive services such as:

- Screenings
- Counseling services
- Preventive medications

The Task Force is made up of 16 volunteer members who serve 4-year terms. Members come from the fields of preventive medicine and primary care, including internal medicine, family medicine, pediatrics, behavioral health, obstetrics and gynecology, and nursing. The Task Force is led by a chair and two vice-chairs. Members are appointed by the Director of the Agency for Healthcare Research and Quality (AHRQ). Members must have no substantial conflicts of interest that could impair the integrity of the work of the Task Force. A list of current USPSTF members, including their biographical information, can be found on the USPSTF Web site (www.USPreventiveServicesTaskForce.org).

Since 1998, through acts of the U.S. Congress, AHRQ has been authorized to convene the Task Force and to provide ongoing scientific, administrative, and dissemination support to the Task Force.

Recommendations

The Task Force makes recommendations to help primary care clinicians and patients decide together whether a preventive service is right for a patient's needs. Its recommendations apply to people who have no signs or symptoms of the specific disease or condition to which a recommendation applies and are for services prescribed, ordered, or delivered in the primary care setting.

Task Force recommendations are based on a rigorous review of existing peer-reviewed evidence. The Task Force assesses the effectiveness of a clinical preventive service by evaluating and balancing the potential benefits and harms of the service. The potential benefits include early identification of disease leading to improvement in health. The potential harms can include adverse effects of the service itself or inaccurate test results that may lead to additional testing, additional risks, or unneeded treatment.

The Task Force does not explicitly consider costs in its assessment of the effectiveness of a service. The Task Force assigns each recommendation a letter grade (A, B, C, or D grade or an I statement) based on the strength of the evidence and on the balance of benefits and harms of the preventive service. More information on USPSTF recommendation grades and a list of all current USPSTF recommendations can be found on the USPSTF Web site.

The Recommendation Making Process

The USPSTF is committed to making its work as transparent as possible. As part of this commitment, the Task Force provides opportunities for the public to provide input during each phase of the recommendation process.

The phases of the topic development process are described below and illustrated in "Steps the USPSTF Takes to Make a Recommendation" at the end of this appendix.

Topic Nomination

The USPSTF considers a broad range of clinical preventive services for its recommendations, focusing on screenings, counseling, and preventive medications. Anyone can nominate a topic for consideration by the Task Force.

Research Plan Development

Once the USPSTF selects a topic for review, it works with an Evidence-based Practice Center (EPC) to develop a draft research plan, which guides the review process and includes key questions and target populations. A draft research plan is posted for public comment, and feedback is incorporated into a final research plan.

Evidence Report and Recommendation Statement Development

Using the final research plan as a guide, the EPC researchers independently gather, review, and analyze evidence on the topic and summarize their findings in a systematic evidence report. The evidence report is sent to subject matter experts for peer review before it is shared with the Task Force.

Then, the entire Task Force discusses and deliberates the evidence, weighs the benefits and harms, and uses the information to determine the effectiveness of a service. The Task Force revises and finalizes a draft recommendation statement based on this discussion.

The draft evidence report and draft recommendation statement are typically posted together on the Task Force Web site for a period of 4 weeks. During the comment period, any member of the public may submit comments on either or both of the documents.

Upon receiving all comments from experts, partners, and the public, the EPC researchers revise the draft evidence report. Once final, the EPC begins to prepare a summary of the evidence report for submission to a peer-reviewed journal.

Final Recommendation Statement

Then, Task Force members review all the comments received and use them to inform the development of the final recommendation statement. The recommendation statement is sent to all Task Force members for final ratification.

The final recommendation statement and evidence summary are published at the same time in a peer-reviewed journal. All recommendation statements and supporting evidence reports are made available on the Task Force Web site (www.USPreventiveServicesTaskForce.org).

Please visit the Task Force Web site to learn how and when to nominate topics for consideration by the Task Force or to comment on topics in development.

Identifying High Priority Research Gaps

In the Patient Protection and Affordable Care Act of 2010, Congress has specifically charged the Task Force with identifying and reporting each year on areas where current evidence is insufficient to make a recommendation on the use of a clinical preventive service, with special attention to those areas where evidence is needed to make recommendations for specific populations and age groups. The USPSTF believes that identifying evidence gaps and highlighting them as priority areas for research will inspire public and private researchers to collaborate and target their efforts to generate new knowledge and address important health priorities. The Annual Report to Congress is available on the Task Force Web site.

Online Resources

On the Task Force Web site, people can:

- View all current USPSTF recommendations, EPC reports, and supporting materials.

- View manuals, slides, videos, and commentaries about the methods and processes the Task Force uses.

- Learn how to interpret recommendations and use them in clinical primary care practice.

- Nominate a new USPSTF member or a topic for a consideration by the Task Force.

- Provide input on specific draft materials during public comment periods.

- Sign up for the USPSTF listserv to receive USPSTF updates.

- Access the Electronic Preventive Services Selector (ePSS), a quick hands-on tool designed to help primary care clinicians and health care teams identify, prioritize, and offer the screening, counseling, and preventive medication services that are appropriate for their patients. The ePSS is available on the Web (epss.ahrq.gov) or as a mobile phone or PDA application.

- Access myhealthfinder. myhealthfinder is a tool for consumers that provides personalized recommendations for preventive services based on the U.S. Preventive Services Task Force; the *Bright Futures* Guidelines; the Centers for Disease Control and Prevention's Advisory Committee on Immunization Practices (ACIP); and the Institute of Medicine's (IOM's) Committee on Preventive Services for Women.

Steps the USPSTF Takes to Make a Recommendation

Create Research Plan

Draft Research Plan
The Task Force works with researchers from an Evidence-based Practice Center (EPC) and creates a draft Research Plan that guides the review process.

Invite Public Comments
The draft Research Plan is posted on the USPSTF Web site for public comment.

Finalize Research Plan
The Task Force and EPC review all comments and address them as appropriate, and the Task Force creates a final Research Plan.

Develop Evidence Report and Recommendation Statement

Draft Evidence Report
Using the final Research Plan, the EPC independently gathers and reviews the available published evidence and creates a draft Evidence Report.

— then —

Draft Recommendation Statement
The Task Force then discusses the draft Evidence Report and the effectiveness of the service. Based on the discussion, the Task Force creates a draft Recommendation Statement.

Invite Public Comments
The draft Evidence Report and draft Recommendation Statement are posted simultaneously on the USPSTF Web site for public comment.

Finalize Evidence Report
The EPC reviews all comments on the draft Evidence Report, addresses them as appropriate, and creates a final Evidence Report.

— then —

Finalize Recommendation Statement
The Task Force discusses the final Evidence Report and any new evidence. The Task Force then reviews all comments on the draft Recommendation Statement, addresses them as appropriate, and creates a final Recommendation Statement.

Disseminate Recommendation Statement

Publish and Disseminate Final Recommendation Statement
The final Recommendation Statement and supporting materials, including the final Evidence Report, are posted on the USPSTF Web site at www.uspreventiveservicestaskforce.org. At the same time, the final Evidence Report and final Recommendation Statement are published together in a peer-reviewed journal. The final Recommendation Statement is also made available through electronic tools and a consumer guide.

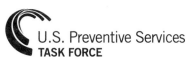

U.S. Preventive Services
TASK FORCE
www.USPreventiveServicesTaskForce.org

More Resources

 ### AHRQ's Improving Primary Care Program

AHRQ's Improving Primary Care Program Web site (www.ahrq.gov/improvingprimarycare) produces evidence and tools to transform the primary care delivery system, resulting in better care, better experiences, and better value. The Program's Web site includes tools, resources, and materials to support health care organizations and engage the entire health care delivery system.

The Program includes two overall project areas with specific areas of focus:

- Improving Primary Care Practice
    - Capacity building
    - Care coordination
    - Clinical-community linkages
    - Health care/system redesign
    - Health information technology integration
    - Behavioral and mental health
    - Primary care practice-based research networks
    - Self-management support
- Evidence-Based Decisionmaking
    - Clinical decision support
    - Multiple chronic conditions
    - Research centers for excellence in clinical preventive services
    - U.S. Preventive Services Task Force

 ### myhealthfinder

A consumer-friendly resource, myhealthfinder (available at www.healthfinder.gov) helps people create a customized list of relevant recommendations for preventive services based on age, sex, and pregnancy status, along with explanations of each recommendation in plain language.

Stay Healthy Brochures

Consumers can use the information in this series of brochures to learn which screening tests you need and when to get them, which medicines may prevent diseases, and daily steps to take for good health. The series includes *Men Stay Healthy at Any Age, Women Stay Healthy at Any Age, Men Stay Healthy at 50+, and Women Stay Healthy at 50+*, all in English and Spanish. Go to http://www.ahrq.gov/patients-consumers/prevention/lifestyle/index.html for the list and choose the title you are interested in.

Community Preventive Services Task Force

Established in 1996 by the U.S. Department of Health and Human Services, the Community Preventive Services Task Force (CPSTF) complements the work of the USPSTF, by addressing preventive services at the community level. The CPSTF assists agencies, organizations, and individuals at all levels (national, State, community, school, worksite, and health care system) by providing evidence-based recommendations about community prevention programs and policies that are effective in saving lives, increasing longevity, and improving Americans' quality of life. The recommendations of the CPSTF are available at www.thecommunityguide.org.

Advisory Committee on Immunization Practices

The Advisory Committee on Immunization Practices, managed and supported by the Centers for Disease Control and Prevention, is a group of medical and public health experts that develops recommendations on how to use vaccines to control diseases in the United States. The recommendations stand as public health advice that will lead to a reduction in the incidence of vaccine preventable diseases and an increase in the safe use of vaccines and related biological products.

The Substance Abuse and Mental Health Services Administration

The Substance Abuse and Mental Health Services Administration provides resources that help health care providers locate and utilize behavioral health services. The Treatment Locator (findtreatment.samhsa.gov) helps find alcohol and drug abuse treatment or mental health treatment

facilities and programs around the country, and the National SBIRT Addiction Technology Transfer Center (ireta.org/ebpsbirt) helps utilize the public health model of screening and counseling to patients on risky or harmful drug and alcohol use.

Healthy People 2020

Healthy People 2020 is an initiative from the U.S. Department of Health and Human Services that challenges individuals, communities, and professionals to take specific steps to ensure good health. Healthy People provides science-based, 10-year national objectives for improving the health of all Americans. Read more at www.healthypeople.gov/2020/default.aspx.

National Guideline Clearinghouse™

A public resource for evidence-based clinical practice guidelines, NGC (guideline.gov/index.aspx) was originally created by AHRQ in partnerships with the American Medical Association and the American Association of Health Plans (now America's Health Insurance Plans). The NGC mission is to provide physicians and other health professionals, health care providers, health plans, integrated delivery systems, purchasers, and others an accessible mechanism for obtaining objective, detailed information on clinical practice guidelines and to further their dissemination, implementation, and use of this information.

Canadian Task Force on Preventive Health Care

The Task Force was established by the Public Health Agency of Canada to develop clinical practice guidelines that support primary care providers in delivering preventive health care. The mandate of the Task Force is to develop and disseminate clinical practice guidelines for primary and preventive care, based on systematic analysis of scientific evidence. Read more at www.canadiantaskforce.ca/.

Cancer Control P.L.A.N.E.T.

A service of the National Cancer Institute, the Cancer Control P.L.A.N.E.T. portal provides access to Web-based resources that can help planners, program staff, and researchers to design, implement, and evaluate evidence-based cancer control programs. Read more at cancercontrolplanet.cancer.gov/index.html.

HealthCare.gov

This Web site (www.healthcare.gov), managed by the U.S. Department of Health and Human Services, helps people take health care into their own hands. It provides information about insurance options, using insurance, the Affordable Care Act, comparing providers, and prevention and wellness—including which preventive services are covered under the Act.

Breast Cancer (2002 Recommendation)*

Title	Screening for Breast Cancer (2002 Recommendation)		
Population	Women ages 40 years and older		
Screening Test	Mammography, with or without clinical breast examination	Clinical breast examination alone	Breast self-examination alone
Recommendation	Screen every 1 to 2 years. Grade: B	No recommendation. Grade: I (Insufficient Evidence)	No recommendation. Grade: I (Insufficient Evidence)

Risk Assessment	Women who are at increased risk for breast cancer (e.g., those with a family history of breast cancer in a mother or sister, a previous breast biopsy revealing atypical hyperplasia, or first childbirth after age 30) are more likely to benefit from regular mammography than women at lower risk.
Screening Tests	There is fair evidence that mammography screening every 12 to 33 months significantly reduces mortality from breast cancer. Evidence is strongest for women ages 50 to 69 years. For women ages 40 to 49 years, the evidence that screening mammography reduces mortality from breast cancer is weaker, and the absolute benefit of mammography is smaller, than it is for older women. Clinicians should refer patients to mammography screening centers with proper accreditation and quality assurance standards to ensure accurate imaging and radiographic interpretation. Clinicians should adopt office systems to ensure timely and adequate follow-up of abnormal results.
Balance of Benefits and Harms	The precise age at which the benefits from screening mammography justify the potential harms is a subjective judgment and should take into account patient preferences. Clinicians should inform women about the potential benefits (reduced chance of dying from breast cancer), potential harms (false-positive results, unnecessary biopsies), and limitations of the test that apply to women their age. The balance of benefits and potential harms of mammography improves with increasing age for women ages 40 to 70 years. Clinicians who advise women to perform breast self-examination or who perform routine clinical breast examination to screen for breast cancer should understand that there is currently insufficient evidence to determine whether these practices affect breast cancer mortality, and that they are likely to increase the incidence of clinical assessments and biopsies.
Other Relevant USPSTF Recommendations	The USPSTF has made recommendations on screening for genetic susceptibility for breast cancer and chemoprevention of breast cancer. These recommendations are available at http://www.uspreventiveservicestaskforce.org/.

*The U.S. Department of Health and Human Services, in implementing the Affordable Care Act, under the standard it sets out in revised Section 2713(a)(5) of the Public Health Service Act, utilizes the 2002 recommendation on breast cancer screening of the U.S. Preventive Services Task Force.

For a summary of the evidence systematically reviewed in making this recommendation, the full recommendation statement, and supporting documents, please go to http://www.uspreventiveservicestaskforce.org/.

Index

Calcium Supplements (see Vitamin D and Calcium Supplementation to Prevent Fractures, Preventive Medication)

Cancer

(see Aspirin or NSAIDS for Prevention of Colorectal Cancer, Preventive Medication)

(see Bladder Cancer, Screening)

(see BRCA-Related Cancer in Women, Screening)

(see Breast Cancer, Preventive Medications)

(see Breast Cancer, Screening)

(see Cervical Cancer, Screening)

(see Colorectal Cancer, Screening)

(see Lung Cancer Screening)

(see Oral Cancer, Screening)

(see Ovarian Cancer, Screening)

(see Prostate Cancer, Screening)

(see Skin Cancer, Counseling)

(see Skin Cancer, Screening)

(see Testicular Cancer, Screening)

---

* indicates new or updated recommendations released March 2012 to March 2014.

Bold text indicates topic of recommendation.

Italic text indicates topic in progress (new or update).

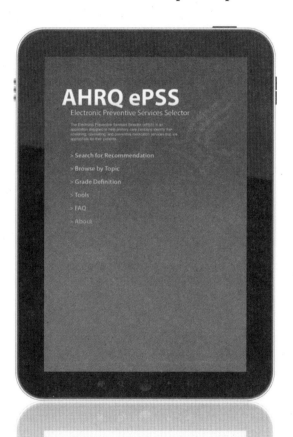